Shared Training and Development Services for Hospitals

Robert A. McGowan
Michael J. Merrill

American Hospital Association
840 North Lake Shore Drive
Chicago, Illinois 60611

AHA

Library of Congress Cataloging in Publication Data

McGowan, Robert A.
    Shared training and development services for
hospitals.

    Includes bibliographical references.
    "AHA catalog no.   "—P.
    1. Hospitals—Staff—In-service training.
2. Medicine—Study and teaching (Continuing
education) 3. Hospitals—Shared services.
I. Merrill, Michael J. II. Title. [DNLM: 1. Hos-
pital shared services. 2. Personnel, Hospital—
Education. 3. Inservice training. WX 18 M478s]
RA972.5.M33 1982   362.1'1'0683   82-8716
ISBN 0-87258-342-2   AACR2

AHA catalog no. 088200

©1982 by the
American Hospital Association
840 North Lake Shore Drive
Chicago, Illinois 60611

3M-8/82-20178

Contents

List of Figures

List of Tables

Foreword

This book presents stages in the process of planning for human resource development (HRD) within the hospital setting and explains the advantages of using a shared-service approach among several hospitals in order to meet increasing HRD needs. The authors, Robert A. McGowan and Michael J. Merrill, assume that the status of the shared service as a tax-exempt or not-for-profit organization, as well as the development of a corporate charter, will have been thoroughly investigated before the project is begun and that appropriate legal counsel will have been consulted.

The book stems from a 1977 National Research Conference on Shared Education Services, sponsored by the Health Education Consortium, Inc. The conference was developed and conducted by the authors, who worked closely with James S. Dolph, director of education for the New England Hospital Assembly. As a result of comments from participants at the conference, the authors realized that a definitive body of work on the topic of shared HRD services was much needed, and set about further formulating and developing their ideas. The result is the present book.

Robert A. McGowan is the president and cofounder of the Institute for Organizational Effectiveness, a professional corporation of consultants offering a variety of management and organizational development services to the hospital and health care industry. He is a former director of the Health Education Consortium, Inc., a shared hospital-based education service in Manchester, NH. He has a broad base of experience as a consultant to hospitals interested in developing internal and multi-institutional human resource development systems.

Michael J. Merrill is an independent group and organizational development consultant with a decade of experience in medical systems. Formerly director of human resources development at University Hospital in Boston, he has had a diverse career as a manager, community development specialist, health systems consultant, and organizational development practitioner. Mr. Merrill's experience in health care organizations ranges from the development of two shared training and development services to complex consulting projects with medical centers. He is a member of NTL Institute, and is affiliated with the consulting firm The Institute, Manchester, NH. Mr. Merrill is also a contributing author to the book *Organizational Development in Health Care Settings.*

Editorial assistance at the AHA was provided by Peg Schultz, assistant editor, and Frank Sabatino, staff editor, under the direction of Marjorie Weissman, manager, Book Department, and Dorothy Saxner, director, Division of Books and Newsletters.

Preface

We are not compromising the truth when we say that dozens of colleagues, administrators, and health care professionals have written this book through us. We want to acknowledge those who stood behind us—in fact and spirit—in our past and present efforts to build and manage effective shared services for training and development.

The New England Hospital Assembly (NEHA) and the New England Hospital and Health Foundation (NEHHF) continually have demonstrated an active and long-term commitment to the development of shared services. We worked for years with James S. Dolph, director of education for NEHA; he provided resources, counsel, support, and hands when we needed them.

Our involvement with Northern Maine Regional Approach to Improved Heath Services through Education (RAISE) and the Manchester Health Education Consortium (HEC) provided the opportunity to develop and test many of the concepts, principles, and techniques described in this book. We thank Research and Education Trust, Inc., of the Maine Hospital Association (MHA) for securing funds provided by Medical Care Development, Inc., a Maine-based organization, to develop RAISE. Christopher Boys, president/chief executive officer of Portsmouth (NH) Hospital and former associate director, MHA, provided strong and visionary leadership. The administrators, health care personnel, and others from Aroostook County, Maine, struggled patiently with us as RAISE developed; without their trust and support, we may not have continued.

The administrators of Manchester (NH) hospitals, Francis Cronin, Dr. Sylvio L. Dupuis, and A. J. St. John, worked with us in developing a similar consortium with a grant from the Veterans Administration. H. Irene Peters, director of education and research, the New Hampshire Hospital Association, was, and is, active in the development of HEC. The staff members, past and present, from RAISE and HEC were valued collaborators, as were the training and development professionals who worked with us. Participants at the 1977 National Research Conference on Shared Education Services will see their stamp in these pages. Several individuals made specific and valuable contributions, among them Timothy Weaver, Ph.D., Lynne Brandon, Ph.D., Janice A. Hughes, and Michael Skaling.

Robert A. McGowan
Michael J. Merrill

Chapter 1

Human Resource Development and the Shared Service Concept

Human Resource Development

Human resource development (HRD) is the conscious, planned process of developing an organization's capabilities to develop and manage human resources to achieve and sustain an optimal level of performance and individual self-esteem. Depending upon whom you talk to and what you read, you will learn that HRD works, does not work, is extremely complex and scientific, defies description, is little more than a passing fad, cannot be evaluated, can always be evaluated, risks becoming professionalized, risks not becoming professionalized, does not really exist, once existed but is now extinct, or is transforming into something else that works. However, the reality is that, broadly defined, HRD is a $100-billion-a-year industry in the United States.

During the past decade, hospitals have expanded their involvement in HRD considerably and with some success. Besides recognizing the need to develop the potential of the personnel they employ, hospitals have also recognized the outside forces that have compelled them to be more attentive to HRD needs. Among these forces are:

- Changing societal values regarding work
- The accelerating obsolescence rate of clinical knowledge
- The labor-intensive nature of health care work as compared with many industrial settings
- Threats of unionism, and the dysfunctional effects unionism has on a health care facility
- A trend toward employee alienation and boredom, often manifesting itself in high absenteeism and turnover, alcohol and drug abuse, and so on
- Dead-end careers in many health care professions
- Increased social and regulatory pressures
- Consumer and regulatory demands for increased efficiency and cost containment
- Requirements for quality assurance and mandatory continuing education
- Burgeoning malpractice litigation
- The recognition that trustees are accountable for their actions

The list could go on, but the point is that, in collaboration with senior management people, HRD professionals have a choice: to proceed in a proactive way to respond to those problems, or to sit tight, doing as little as possible for the moment, hoping the problems will abate.

Components of an HRD Program

The components of an HRD system include:

- Management and supervisory development, especially executive education, middle-management development, and first-line supervisory development
- Assessment training, often through a presupervisory assessment program
- Nursing education, including clinical skills training, new product usage, interpersonal skills development, and degree programs
- Orientation processes, for example, new employee training, new graduate internship, and registered nurse refresher training
- Upward mobility training, such as clerical/secretarial training, GED high school equivalency opportunities, medical secretary training, and career development training
- Career development training, including career counseling and planning, educational and occupational referral, and tuition assistance
- Nonnursing staff development and training, such as on-the-job training for support personnel and technical training for ancillary service workers
- Professional development for HRD staff, especially training for trainers, cultivation of consulting skills, and organizational development
- Physician education
- Trustee education
- Community and patient education
- Other opportunities, such as availability of audiovisual resources
- Manpower planning
- Multicultural development/affirmative action plan

Meeting HRD needs, which will increase in intensity in the 1980s and 1990s, is a tall order for any single institution, no matter how well managed or financed. At present, some health care organizations ignore many of these needs or approach them piecemeal. We are arguing for an approach that moves from fragmentation toward integration, from goal confusion toward goal agreement, from split resources toward shared resources, and from cost ineffectiveness toward cost effectiveness. The challenge is to do this *without* compromising the identity of any institution or limiting the freedom of choice of executives and human resources professionals who must respond in a unique way to pressing internal needs that may not be shared by other institutions.

The Shared HRD Service

One way to meet the various HRD needs of an institution is through a shared HRD service. A shared HRD service is an organizational arrangement created by two or more health care providers banding together to gain economies of scale, improvements in quality, or increased political power through the sharing of selected services or joint projects.

Adopting this general definition allows latitude in the design and implementation of shared services. The point is that the definition must not be allowed to close off potentialities. For example, one definition, that shared services (or consortiums) are membership organizations with full-time staff devoted to joint planning and programming, forecloses arrangements in which full-time staffing is not a valid choice.

The task of this book is to share ways to meet pressing human resource development needs. We are challenging you to consider using the organizational form called a shared service to address the HRD needs of your organization and to devise alternative ways to manage and develop human resources. This book is based on our experiences with shared services as internal and external consultants, on the learning and the reports of our fellow travelers in similar ventures across the country, and on the National Research Conference on Shared Education Services cosponsored by the

New England Hospital Assembly and the Manchester Health Education Consortium in April 1977.

At the conference, representatives from 21 shared service organizations met for three days to assess the state of the art, including various models that have been developed, benefits and limitations, major barriers to initiation, successful strategies, tools, programs developed, and so on, and to examine each organization in depth.[1] Prior to the conference, each participant responded in writing to the following questions:

- What are the five most critical problems you confronted, or are facing, in the development of your organization? Describe the steps that you took, or are taking, to overcome each problem.
- What are the three most outstanding benefits and limitations of shared services that you would share with a colleague or with an administrator?
- What are four positive outcomes of your shared service that resulted in concrete improvements in the effectiveness of participating organizations.
- What conditions do you believe must be met to develop a successful shared venture?
- What are the three things that you have learned from your project that you think would be most useful to other participants in the conference?
- What are the three most important things that you hope to learn at the conference?

Each participant presented a paper at the conference that highlighted certain aspects of his or her organization, and each shared service was discussed at length. Structured exercises were also conducted, during which participants shared their combined knowledge and experience by generating lists in response to the following questions:

- What are your "five noble truths" about the organization and operation of shared services efforts?
- What is your ideal picture of a shared service (include how it is organized, what is happening, and what people are doing) in an urban environment? Repeat the process for a rural environment.
- What programs have you developed that you are willing to share/sell?
- What are the most significant things that your shared service has accomplished that you would like to brag about?
- What are the indicators that a shared service is too large or too small?

By the end of the conference, the group had a much clearer understanding of the various models that have been developed, as well as benefits and limitations, major barriers to initiation, successful strategies, tools, programs developed, and so on. Although we believe that these organizations were fairly representative of the range of shared service models, we recognize that the future of shared service will rest on the imagination and resources of its proponents.

Shared Services: State of the Art

A decade ago, the state of the art in the development of shared services was but a few years beyond primitive; today, such multi-institutional efforts are almost commonplace.

The following statement clearly indicates the strong support of multi-institutional arrangements among hospitals in order to meet various needs.[2]

> The (hospital) institution should be aware of program decisions of neighboring institutions and of other proposed new programs in the community pertaining to health care services, facilities, health education and manpower development. It should recognize its interdependence with other health organizations and community groups with health interests and encourage continual creative interaction.

Because there are limited resources upon which to call, hospitals should participate with other institutions to distribute effectively those limited resources and, where resources are inadequate, to develop programs for raising additional funds.

AHA Survey Data

The "Hospital Shared Services Participation Profile," compiled in 1978 by the American Hospital Association's Hospital Data Center, indicated that 80 percent of the 5,742 U.S. registered hospitals responding to an AHA survey were participating in at least one shared service activity.[3] The following findings can be learned from the report:

- The most frequently mentioned shared service was purchasing, particularly for medical-surgical supplies, intravenous solutions, drugs, dietary, and linen services; 80 percent of those sharing services reported that they were satisfied with the service.
- Hospitals were most interested in developing shared services in the areas of biomedical/clinical engineering, printing and duplicating, microfilms, laundry and linen, and audiovisual equipment.
- Large institutions tended to share more than did small ones; for example, 92 percent of hospitals with 400 to 499 beds shared services.

Table 1, below, provides a summary of data about shared HRD services, or interest in developing them.

Depending on the number of beds per hospital, a range of 9 to 22 percent of hospitals surveyed shared one or more HRD services, and satisfaction rates range from 78 to 85 percent. However, few hospitals seemed interested in exploring the development of shared HRD services. Trusting the data at face value, one might conclude that only 158 hospitals (2.8 percent of those surveyed) are interested in sharing management training services, that 169 hospitals (2.9 percent) are interested in nursing services, and so on. Does this mean that the potential market for the development of shared HRD services is small, that the apparent lack of interest is low because hospitals do not understand or value HRD, or that hospitals cannot envision the development of such services on a shared basis? Our belief is that the market is sometimes perceived as small because hospitals tend not to attach a high priority to HRD and, at times, are not confident that they can, or should, develop such services on a shared basis.

Organizational Models

A variety of models for shared HRD services, ranging from the simple to the complex, have emerged to seek the benefits while minimizing the limitations. Each

Table 1. Data on Survey of 5,742 Hospitals

Service	Interested in HRD Service Number	%	Involved in HRD Service Number	%	Satisfied with Existing HRD Service Number	%
Clerical education and training	408	8.9	115	2.0	332	81.4
Management training	806	17.5	158	2.8	670	83.1
Nursing education	1,014	22.0	169	2.9	849	83.7
Audiovisual equipment	754	16.4	202	3.5	644	85.4
Management engineering	738	16.0	158	2.8	602	81.6
Personnel/collective bargaining	634	13.8	58	1.0	496	78.2
Other	585	12.7	169	1.2	498	85.1

model is influenced by its specific goals and objectives, funding sources, and history in relationship to the individual or agencies that assume responsibility for initiating the project. The most common organizational arrangements include:

- Independent not-for-profit organizations offering membership and/or contracted services to individual hospitals within a region (the services are generally limited to HRD activities, and the focus of the services provided is determined by number of organizations)
- Special projects of state or regional hospital associations, generally initiated as the result of the award of a grant from a foundation or the federal government
- Formal education institutions (colleges and universities) offering specific education and training services for hospitals with structured provider input into the decision-making process
- Contractual relationships among individual hospitals for specific programs that are to be developed jointly by pooling resources, by the staff of one individual hospital, or by an external source
- Centralized programs, cosponsored by individual institutions, that bring in educational institutions or private consultants as resources
- Multihospital corporations with a centralized HRD function
- HRD staff working for state or regional hospital associations who either coordinate centralized education experiences or provide specific services for individual institutions
- Individual hospitals offering internal programs that are open to participation by others

Although there are many pure examples of these models, most shared HRD services are variants or hybrids of the basic arrangements.

Funding Mechanisms

As might be expected, there is an equal diversity of cooperative HRD funding mechanisms. Most complex efforts began with some form of funding from private foundations or the federal government. Success ultimately depends upon independent funding, however, and the various funding sources include membership assessment, program income, and the marketing of educational programs and materials. Membership assessment provides the largest percentage of funding, and the various formulas for determining membership assessment take into consideration the number of beds, the number of staff, the operating budget, a percentage of gross revenue, a percentage of association dues, and a simple standard assessment of all members. The approaches to charges for educational programs include no charge for member hospitals but fees for nonmembers, reduced rates for member hospitals, no registration fee for members but full reimbursement for printed material, and special bulk rates for attendance at large numbers of programs.

Common Shared Services

The most common forms of shared HRD services fall into the following categories:

- Technical training—Educational programs for hospital personnel, including nurses, social workers, laboratory and x-ray personnel, medical secretaries, infection control officers, occupational and physical therapists, financial managers, and others, most daylong workshops offered either by the staff of member institutions or by private consultants
- Management training programs—Top, middle, and first-line management training programs, including centralized programs offered by private consultants, package programs purchased for internal use, programs developed by staff of the shared service, and programs developed by staff within individual member organizations

- Core technical programs—Programs ranging from 20 to 60 hours in length, including coronary care, respiratory care, medical terminology, nursing aide training, pharmacology, and others, many for the purpose of formal certification
- Physician education programs—Programs generally offered on a weekly basis and approved for medical staff continuing education credit, usually conducted by medical staff of the member hospitals or by speakers with a national or international reputation
- Trustee education programs—Programs generally conducted on a centralized basis for trustees from member institutions, frequently using speakers with national reputations on health care issues

Examples of support services offered by various shared HRD services include coordination of education activities through some form of monthly calendar; a resource clearinghouse to facilitate sharing of training resources including audiovisual hardware and software; training materials, library materials, and other learning resources; and advocacy for member hospitals with external education institutions to bring their resources in programs to member hospitals, thus reducing cost for travel, room, and board.

Staffing Patterns

Staffing patterns for shared service range from full-time staff, limited use of member hospital staff, and external consultants hired for specific programs, to a mix of all three. Those shared services that hire full-time staff generally experience a higher level of success, and they are more likely to become permanent. At the same time, however, when full-time staff are hired, there is a danger that hiring full-time staff will stifle creative ways to share existing staff and that internal resources will be undeveloped, thereby reducing the effectiveness of the shared services effort. The maximum payoff from shared HRD services comes from the sharing of the unique talents and expertise that are within each hospital. But this is often a difficult task because of feelings of competition, concerns about equity, and differences in policies, procedures, styles, and so on.

Advantages and Disadvantages

One of the clearest advantages of shared services is that hospitals are able to pool their resources and hire professionals with a broader range of sophisticated skills. A number of shared services have succeeded in hiring individuals who have extensive experience in organizational development and human resource development. Shared services are also able to offer member institutions services often beyond the financial reach of any single institution, such as organizational assessment, strategic planning, senior management team development, crisis intervention, consultation to individual managers, and other activities related to improving organizational effectiveness. Yet AHA data and the findings of the National Research Conference on Shared Education Services also indicate that, although shared HRD services are seen as beneficial by participants, such services also present certain limitations. Participants at the conference developed the following lists of benefits and limitations.

Advantages of a shared HRD service are as follows:
- More effective HRD services
- More sophisticated programs to meet the demands of technological and knowledge explosions
- Access to the services of skilled HRD professionals, which one hospital could not afford
- Increased access to HRD resources of other institutions
- Allows for more specialization, building on the strengths of member institutions

- More effective use of existing HRD personnel
- Reduction in costly duplication of resources, personnel, and programs
- Higher probability of receiving grants and other sources of revenue
- Strengthens "provider" input into education institutions
- Increased ability to develop a better data base to identify needs and trends in HRD

On the other hand, the following are seen as limitations of a shared HRD service:

- Competition between both service and education providers
- Power/control issues
- Varying organizational philosophies and priorities resulting in not meeting everyone's top priority needs
- Inequities in resources between member organizations resulting in an imbalance of "in-kind" contributions
- Lack of effective internal education systems in member organizations, resulting in "underuse" by some
- "Significant" time commitment required of senior and middle managers
- In larger geographical areas, greater difficulty in developing cohesiveness

Making Shared Services Work

Recognizing the hard realities of making a shared HRD service work, the participants in the 1977 National Research Conference identified the following seven criteria for successful shared services:

1. A firm commitment to education and training on the part of the administrators of member institutions
2. A clearly defined decision-making process
3. Sufficient preliminary work prior to any commitment to sort out the function of the venture, often facilitated by an external consultant
4. Extensive involvement of the target population, especially middle managers in the planning process
5. A sound financial base (meaning hard money)
6. A systematic approach to planning, organizing, and controlling the process
7. Full-time or part-time staff

Posture of the CEO

The posture of the chief executive officer toward HRD may be the single most important influence determining the extent to which and how successfully a hospital involves itself in HRD activities. The reason for this, and the reason why a firm commitment to education and training by administrators is listed as the first criterion of a successful venture, can be understood by exploring what is known as the "disincentive process."

The following elements comprise the disincentive process:[4]

- The benefits of HRD are not clear to top management.
- Top management rarely evaluates and rewards managers and supervisors for carrying out effective HRD.
- Top management rarely plans and budgets systematically for HRD.
- Managers usually do not account for HRD in service delivery.
- Supervisors have difficulty meeting productions norms with employees in HRD.
- Therefore, supervisors and managers train and develop employees unsystematically and mostly for short-term objectives.
- Behavioral and project objectives of HRD are often imprecise.
- HRD programs external to the agency sometimes teach techniques and methods contrary to practices of the participant's organization.
- Timely information about external HRD training programs is often difficult to obtain.

- HRD effectiveness is impaired as a result of statutory restrictions on travel funds.
- The HRD professional provides limited counseling and consulting services to the rest of the organization.

Simply summarized, the disincentive process asserts that if the benefits of HRD are clear to top management, and if top management rewards HRD behavior and plans and budgets for HRD activities, then HRD can contribute directly to organizational needs. If the benefits are not clear to top management, minimal payoff, at best, and disaster, at worst, can be expected. Thus, any attempt to build a shared HRD service must break the cycle of disincentives. The model presented in chapter 2 deals with this reality.

Assessing Your CEO's HRD Posture

A quick test that will help you pinpoint your CEO's HRD posture is shown in figure 1, below.[5] Simply answer each question yes or no. If you or your CEO can answer yes to 16 or more questions, your organization is heavily committed to HRD; if you answer yes to 12 or more, your organization sees HRD as more than a luxury; if you answer yes to 10 or less, your organization probably sees HRD as irrelevant to meeting organizational goals. This quick test can give an indication of the degree of

---

Does your CEO:

1. Take an active part in deciding what the hospital's development activities will be?
2. Have a clear, concise philosophy to manage by, to expect others to manage by, and to communicate to new managers?
3. Participate in a training or development activity each year?
4. Extend his or her involvement in your organization's training programs beyond kick-off speeches and "well done" wrap-ups?
5. Have a budget allocation for his or her own professional and personal development?
6. Make time to talk about human resources development plans with his or her management team?
7. Actively work to develop a successor?
8. Consider the head of your HRD department (or counterpart) part of his or her management team?
9. Ever consider putting a key manager in charge of the hospital's HRD?
10. Have any HRD persons on a list of "high potential" persons?
11. Know who the top personnel developer in the organization is?
12. Reward a good manager for developing other good managers?
13. Personally conduct performance appraisals at least four times a year?
14. Allow managers to rate their subordinates' performance as they see it rather than demand a statistically even distribution of ratings? (If not, he or she has no performance appraisal system, only a salary review system.)
15. Know, without looking it up, who is in charge of managing the hospital's HRD activities?
16. Talk with the top HRD person regularly (once per month)?
17. Allow the chief HRD support person direct access to him or her?
18. Consider the chief HRD support person to be an organizational change agent?
19. Ask persons (all of them) how they feel about their jobs and the company more than once every three years?
20. If you asked a line manager to become your training or HRD manager, would he or she consider that appointment an opportunity rather than a punishment?

Adapted, with permission, from the October 1976 issue of TRAINING, The Magazine of Human Resources Development. Copyright 1976, Lakewood Publications, Minneapolis, MN (612)333-0471. All rights reserved.

Figure 1. Assessment of a CEO's HRD Posture

support to be expected from a CEO if the development of a shared HRD service is contemplated.

One administrator of a metropolitan teaching hospital views the HRD function in the following way:

> Because the health care industry and health care organizations will become more involved in multihospital systems, or "megasystems," to realize economies of scale, the role of the HRD profession will change. The HRD function must become more proactive in anticipating and acting to meet critical HRD needs, becoming the eyes and ears of the CEO on human resource issues, and prepare to change and adapt while helping others, including managers and clinicians, to do the same.[6]

This is the view of an administrator who would score 16 to 18 on the test.

Summary

HRD is often misunderstood and is a relatively new concept in the health care industry. But a body of experience, literature, and research that demonstrates the impact effective HRD can have on a health care organization is beginning to emerge. *The Journal of Applied Behavioral Sciences* recently published a special issue on organizational change efforts in health care settings.[7] Health care journals such as *Hospitals* and *Trustee* are becoming more attentive to HRD issues. Individual institutions, for example, the Kaiser-Permanente System, University Hospital in Boston, and Greater Southeast Community Hospital in Washington, DC, have successfully built solid HRD efforts. Shared service organizations such as the Manchester Health Education Consortium (New Hampshire), Regional In-Service Education (RISE) (Maine), the Maryland Health Education Institute, and dozens of others have launched highly sophisticated educational and developmental efforts to improve the abilities of their members to function in a changing world.

We contend, then, that the best strategy of good human resources development, whether in a shared service or a single institution, is not to be a risk taker, but to be so thorough and imaginative that you eliminate risk and yet can do dramatic things. This book attends to that advice; we will outline a process that is thorough, trusting you to use imagination to find your own path.

Obviously, the development of a shared HRD service able to effectively address needs in each of the areas discussed in this chapter approaches the ideal. We know of no shared service or health care institution that can claim a system so comprehensive. Thus, the developers of a shared HRD service face two tasks: (1) to select those areas in which HRD needs are most critical to the long-term and short-term objectives of the institution and (2) to decide which needs to address through a shared service and which to pursue internally. Numerous configurations could emerge; one shared service may choose to build a comprehensive system to address all, or many, HRD needs; another might focus on a single area such as management education or trustee education; a third may find several areas in which sharing is the feasible alternative. The point is to find the right mix so that each set of needs is dealt with in the most effective and efficient manner. How to make those choices is explained in chapter 3.

NOTES

1. Participants included representatives from Area Health Education Consortium for Southeast Nebraska; American Society for Heathcare Education and Training of the American Hospital Association, Chicago; Central Minnesota Area Health Education Consortium, St. Cloud, MN; Eastern Carolina Health Education System, Florence, SC; Elizabeth (NJ) Hospital; Greater Cleveland Hospital Association; Health Central Institute, Minneapolis; Hospital Consortium, Fort Dodge, IA; Human Services Development Institute, University of

Maine, Portland-Gorham, Portland; James Mercy Hospital, Hornell, NY; Manchester Health Education Consortium, Manchester, NH; Maryland Hospital Education Institute, Lutherville; the Massachusetts Hospital Association, Burlington, MA; Mount Auburn Hospital, Cambridge, MA; New England Hospital Assembly Incorporated, Durham, NH; New England Hospital and Health Foundation, Inc., Durham, NH; Northern Maine RAISE, Presque Isle, ME; Pee Dee Area Health Education Center, Florence, SC; Project RISE, Waterville, ME; University Hospital, Boston; Wesley Medical Center, Wichita, KS.

2. Cochrane, J. D., and Fourkas, T., editors. *Hospital Consortia.* Sacramento, CA: California Hospital Association, 1979.

3. American Hospital Association. "Hospital Shared Services Participation Profile." Unpublished report, Hospital Data Center of the American Hospital Association, 1978.

4. United States Civil Service Commission. Disincentives to Effective Employee Training and Development. Washington, DC: Government Printing Office, 1967.

5. The chief executive's role in human resources development. *Training.* 13:23, Oct. 1976.

6. Conversation with author.

7. See *Journal of Applied Behavioral Sciences,* vol. 14, no. 3, entire issue, 1978.

Chapter 2

Stages in the Development of a Shared Service

Model for Shared Service Development

Whenever different institutions attempt to integrate organizations or services to achieve common or negotiated goals, they will face a number of dilemmas:[1]

- *What are the goals of the shared service?* To improve efficiency, effectiveness, or both? To compete or collaborate with nonmember institutions? To encourage growth or achieve stabilization?
- *Will shared services build trust or maintain distrust?* That is, will a shared service help its members build the trust necessary to achieve a desired integration of services, or will it simply allow each to keep its autonomy while keeping the distrust within tolerable limits?
- *Are shared services really more efficient?* A shared service may increase efficiency, such as in the training of coronary/intensive care nursing personnel, but will it achieve needed change? Can hospitals tolerate a period of inefficiency as the shared service builds the expertise and commitment to truly make a difference?
- *Which viewpoint prevails, the institutional or coalitional?* Will some institutional identity be compromised in order to achieve the goals of the coalition? Can the shared service work in a situation characterized by high autonomy while pursuing joint goals?

To resolve these and other issues, shared service organizers must find a way to negotiate a complex and tortuous course of development. Numerous writers have proposed models for developing shared service organizations.[1,2,3] Each model has its merits, but leaves some questions begging. Therefore, we chose to develop our own model, one that incorporates the best of each of these, captures our experience, and builds on the learning from the National Research Conference on Shared Education Services discussed in chapter 1.

The 17-step model, displayed in figure 2, page 12, depicts our sense of how a shared service develops, a process that key actors can manage in order to achieve the results they seek. The model proceeds through four stages: preaffiliation, formation, implementation, and stabilization/renewal. Each stage includes an outcome and one or two decision points. For example, the outcome of stage 2 is that institutions reach an agreement to organize a shared service and approve institutional involvement in the venture.

A strong feature of this model is that it focuses on both the institutional and the interinstitutional levels. We view the development of a shared service as an interplay between the needs, readiness, motivations, and long-range plans of a single institu-

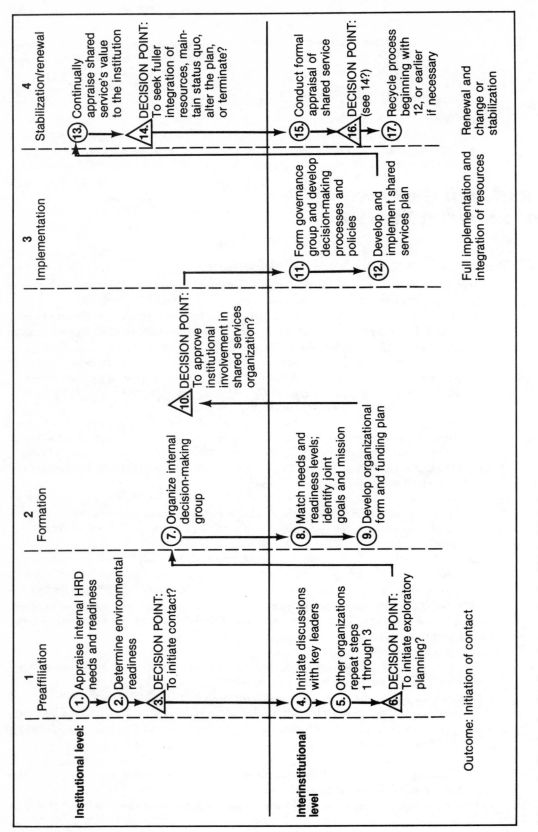

Figure 2. Stages in the Development of a Shared Service

tion and its potential partners in a multi-institutional coalition. The model exemplifies the careful planning that must be done inside an institution's walls as well as in the collaborative domain. Chapters 3 through 6 provide a walk-through of the model, step by step and stage by stage, allowing you the opportunity to apply the concepts to your own situation.

Preaffiliation

The preaffiliation stage begins when a single institution or decision maker perceives a need that may be met in some cooperative venture. This ends when that institution and others agree to initiate exploratory planning, or aborts when either party decides that further action should not be taken at that time. The ultimate question here is: Who should join the venture? At the institutional level, there are three steps in the preaffiliation stage.

1. Appraise internal HRD needs and readiness. This diagnostic step requires that an institution assess its HRD needs and decide how ready it is to tackle those needs in a cooperative manner with other institutions.
2. Determine environmental readiness. A host of factors in the environment can serve to enable or disable a shared service venture in its developmental process. During this step, an individual institution can look at these forces and decide whether they are manageable.
3. DECISION POINT: To initiate contact with other institutions? If the data in step 2 suggest that the forces in the environment are conducive to shared services development, and if the institution is ready internally, then a single institution can decide to initiate a contact with other institutions for mutual exploration. If this situation is not present, an institution can choose to drop, postpone, or reassess the situation.

At the interinstitutional level, preaffiliation is composed of these stages, steps 4 through 6.

4. Initiate discussions with key leaders. The initiating institution introduces the idea to others in an attempt to establish a dialog.
5. Other organizations repeat steps 1-3. If other organizations are interested they can repeat the first three steps.
6. DECISION POINT: To initiate exploratory planning? Once each institution has assessed the internal and external situations, the group can agree to pursue the possibilities more formally.

Formation

The formation stage begins with the tentative commitment to explore mutual interests. It ends when institutions agree to integrate resources in a shared service, or aborts when one or more institutions choose not to proceed, for whatever reasons. The key question in stage 2 is: Do we become a member? At the institutional level, the formation phase contains a single step.

7. Organize an internal decision-making group. The task of this group is to manage the internal planning process and to coordinate efforts with the interinstitutional process.

At the interinstitutional level, the institutions must:

8. Match needs and readiness levels, and identify a mission and goals. This process is designed to determine how well individual needs and readiness levels fit together and whether that fit is defined clearly enough to proceed with planning. If so, the next step is to carefully develop a mission statement and agree on goals. The outcome of this step is to define the function of the shared services organization.
9. Develop the organizational form. With the function clearly defined, the next

step is to create an appropriate structure, one that will enable the new coalition to maximize its investment and achieve its goals It is critical not to complete this step until step 8 is accomplished.

Then, each institution reaches a decision point:

10. DECISION POINT: To approve institutional involvement in the proposed organization? At this point, decision usually comes easily; the organization is now in a better position to understand more clearly how the proposed shared service will affect its operations and long-range plans.

Implementation

The implementation stage involves internal activity and emphasizes joint planning among participating institutions. The obvious question in the implementation stage is: How do we get things done? This stage ends when the shared service succeeds in implementing a well-conceived plan. Critical steps in the implementation phase are listed below.

11. Form a governance group, and develop decision-making processes and operating policies. This is difficult, detailed work, but in the end it produces the cement that holds the day-to-day operation together. Governing a multi-institutional organization is a taxing business, and the dynamics of doing so need to be carefully considered here.

12. Develop and implement the shared services plan. The plan needs to be as well defined as the governance structure and the decision-making process. It is critical that key actors from each institution be involved here and that the task not be delegated downward in the organization.

Stabilization and Renewal

During the stabilization and renewal stage, the shared service enters a continual process of appraisal and planning. The question for the final stage is: How will we grow? Each institution should:

13. Continually appraise the shared service's value to the institution. Required in this step is the existence of an internal mechanism for ongoing appraisal, one that provides the data for future planning.

14. DECISION POINT: Seek fuller integration of resources, maintain the status quo, alter the plan, or terminate? Any of these decisions may be appropriate. The point is to have the institution crystallize its own sense of progress so that it can enter a dialog with other institutions about the future of the shared service. It is important to be able to respond in a responsible and timely manner, because needs and circumstances change so quickly.

At the interinstitutional level, the shared service governance group needs to:

15. Conduct a formal appraisal of the shared services effort. Although each institution has done its own internal appraisal, a joint discussion brings fuller perspective.

16. DECISION POINT: (repeat step 14?) The governance group revises its future in this step.

17. Recycle process at step 12 (earlier if necessary). If the governance group decides to renew or change itself, there will be a need to redefine the mission and goals and develop a new operating plan; if the status quo is maintained, there may be a need only for fine tuning.

If the process seems cumbersome, it may be because building a shared service is a difficult proposition. Nonetheless, our research on the development operation and the impact of a shared service indicates that many failed attempts would have succeeded if these steps were followed.

Planned Change

When you attempt to build a shared service, you are committing yourself to a demanding involvement in planned change. You should keep in mind the following caveats based on research done on planned change:[4]

- Change is not likely to occur unless there is a real *need* to change, if there is something that creates real concern. Plans for change should deal with the important issues where there is some commitment to wanting to improve.
- Change occurs most readily if supported by respected authorities or others. If those who are highly respected do not support the change effort, it is not likely to succeed. Respected formal and informal leaders should be included in the change program so they will lend their support.
- Change occurs most readily if people are involved in the change planning and implementation rather than having the change imposed on them.
- Change is more likely to succeed if people can clearly see that the change will result in an improvement of their situation, will result in greater rewards and self-esteem, and will allow their own and organizational goals to be achieved.
- Change is more likely to result if the planning is specific rather than general. Plans for change must identify clearly and specifically who is to do what, at what time.

This research confirms many principles covering support, communication, sequenced activities, clarity of purpose, organizational integrity, and contingency planning that were developed in the 1977 National Research Conference on Shared Education Services (see chapter 1).

Support

There is a close relationship between the level of organizational support and the ongoing development of the system. Shared HRD services are very complex, and little progress will be made without strong support from all levels of the organization. The manner in which each step of the model is implemented and managed will have an impact on building support that should continue to deepen as the process develops.

Involve the right people in the process from the very beginning. It is essential to identify the key actors that should be on board at the beginning of the process, how you want them to be involved, and what type of support you need from them during the initial stages of the process.

Tune in to what the key people and organizations are looking for and move to meet their needs whenever possible. The fact that each organization involved in a shared education service has a unique set of strengths and weaknesses means that each also will have very different priorities. It is important to clarify the priorities of each member organization so that they can be addressed.

Keep in touch with the informal leaders. Leadership is not simply a function of one's position or membership in key decision-making groups. Many other people who have a great deal of informal power and influence exist within the system, including union leaders, self-appointed change agents, persuasive people, and so on. If support is going to be developed that will enhance the development of the project, recognition of informal leaders and development of their support is critical.

Communication

Be straight with people. People will develop a much higher level of trust and be more willing to provide support if they know that they are receiving an honest picture of the pros and cons, the benefits and limitations, and the potential problems and risks that might be expected. Too often planners paint the rosy side of the picture; when things go awry, bad feelings result, and support is withdrawn.

Provide feedback to all members of the organization regarding progress in the system. Visibility is an important issue in developing and maintaining support for shared efforts.

Avoid surprises. Any multi-institutional effort provides an opportunity to act on overt and covert agendas. It is important to be clear about what the shared service is doing, especially when particular changes or activities might have an impact on an organization or department. No one likes to be caught by surprise; persons who are surprised usually attempt to defend themselves because they are not quite sure what is happening.

Sequenced Activities

The real world seldom follows logical sequences when implementing programs. The model implies that the steps should be implemented in the sequence indicated. Although we believe that this is true, the needs, priorities, and objectives of member organizations will vary. It is certainly legitimate, therefore, to start at any place on the model as a strategy for developing initial support. If the effort is to be effective over the long run, however, significant energy must be be invested in each step of the model. For example, proceeding very far with program development without defining the mission of the organization, assessing needs, or establishing objectives could lead to failure.

Start with activities that result in tangible progress and worthwhile achievements. Many shared education services are looked upon with skepticism during their initial stages. This attitude will prevail until concrete results are delivered. Thus, early programming should be designed to achieve success. The more complex issues can be addressed later on as support develops within the system.

Whenever possible, focus on critical problems (such as injuries, infections, turnover) that could save the organization money, or on problems that are recognized most clearly by the administration and the staff. Pressures for cost containment and increased productivity in hospitals are real, and HRD ought to play a role in responding to these pressures.

Make use of the data presently available, such as surveys, audits, and so forth, to identify problems. Hospital personnel are surveyed to death and these activities ought to be kept to a minimum. Plenty of data are already available in most institutions produced by various audits, surveys, and other types of studies. Before conducting new surveys, these data should be culled for relevant information. It is also important to pay close attention to how much of what kind of information is made available by the various institutions. Access to information is a major indicator of the level of support and trust.

Clarity of Purpose

Be clear about what the project is going to do, what you expect the results to be, and what it will cost. A common belief in many hospital organizations is that it is impossible to measure output. Educators are inclined to make similar statements. Although it is true that many aspects of education, training, and development are hard to evaluate in concrete terms, there are ways to measure outcome. If support for shared HRD services is expected, what the services will accomplish, within what time frame, and at what cost should be predicted with some degree of accuracy. Without this information, it becomes very difficult for administrators to decide whether or not to participate.

Organizational Integrity

Work with member organizations and not for them. Education and training is a responsibility of the entire organization and its managers, not just the HRD function.

Internal education functions are constantly at risk of being delegated and those charged with this specific responsibility often end up relatively powerless. It is important to keep the responsibility for development of employees with the organization and the individual managers involved and to help these individuals address that responsibility in an effective manner.

Keep the structure of the shared service as simple as its mission allows.

Contingency Planning

Develop conscious strategies to overcome barriers. No effort to develop a shared HRD service can be managed without running into barriers and pitfalls; this is a normal part of any organizational change process. Rather than viewing these barriers as negative forces, participants should view them as opportunities to develop the system. The secret is to develop game plans, or strategies, for dealing with the barriers that apply the aforementioned principles and that avoid win/lose confrontations.

A key feature of the model discussed in this chapter is the leadership demands placed upon key actors in a collaborative effort. A shared HRD organization can be a complex undertaking, one that demands a variety of leadership tasks and skills to guide the formal or informal alliance through its developmental and operational stages. The central question is: What leadership tasks and skills are involved and required at this particular stage in the development of a shared HRD service? The participants at the 1977 conference on shared services confirmed this need as they explored the relationship between leadership effectiveness and style and the relative success or failure of the shared service. Thus, leadership was viewed as the key variable in a shared service venture. A corollary question is: How do I, as a leader of my own organization, resolve the inevitable conflict between my interests and those of the shared service?[5] As each stage is discussed in detail in the following chapters, the different leadership tasks and skills required will be highlighted in an attempt to provide a fluid structure that recognizes the contingencies forced on it by the environment.

NOTES

1. Starkweather, D. Issues of motivation for management and governance. In: *Hospital Consortia,* edited by J. D. Cochrane and T. Fourkas, pp. 114-29. Sacramento, CA: California Hospital Association, 1979.

2. American Hospital Association. A guide to shared educational services. *Hospitals, J.A.H.A.* 49:73, Aug. 1, 1975.

3. A model was developed by Behavioral Sciences Resources, Inc., Provo, UT, and shared with the authors.

4. Sheldon, A., and Barrell, D. The Janus principle. *Health Care Manage. Rev.* Spring 1977.

5. Weisbord, M. *Organizational Diagnosis: A Workbook of Theory and Practice.* Reading, MA: Addison-Wesley Pub. Co., 1978. p. 4.

Chapter 3

The Preaffiliation Stage

Diagnosis precedes the treatment of a patient. Treatment does not begin without a diagnosis. This principle should be extended to the world of administration, organization, and HRD. Yet planners often embark on new ventures without an adequate diagnosis of the problem. Experience dictates the obvious: the effective development of a shared HRD service hinges on a clear and painstaking diagnosis of the strengths and weaknesses of this approach in solving perceived problems. If the outcome of the preaffiliation stage is to decide to initiate contact with others who may want to develop a shared HRD service, valid data are needed with which to make an informed choice about the feasibility of such an undertaking.

Diagnosis can be defined as an active process of determining:

- What is the situation or state of affairs today?
- What ought to be the situation at some future time?
- How is the gap closed between what is and what ought to be?

In some ways, the planner is like an air traffic controller who sits in front of a radar screen and interprets blips. To a well-trained observer, those blips communicate an enormous amount of critical information about whether an aircraft is on or off course, if there is danger of collision or close calls, what traffic patterns exist, and so forth. Making a diagnosis about whether to develop a shared service is a similar process. The planner's task is to identify signals that exist in the hospital environment.

The diagnostic process is continuous, recycling itself as a shared service passes through its developmental stages and alters its form in response to contingencies. An action research model, depicted in figure 3, page 20, summarizes the process.[1] The administrator of a single institution senses that his or her organization's HRD needs are not being addressed adequately and that some form of shared service might help. The administrator conceives a study, introduces it to those who need to be involved, gathers and collates data, and relays that data back to key decision makers. If appropriate, those people may choose to plan a course of action, implement the plan, and follow up on the results.The process is repeated as decision makers scan for new problems and challenges. A critical feature of the action research model is that those who will make decisions and those who will be most affected by them are involved.

The action research model underlies the 17-step model proposed in chapter 2.

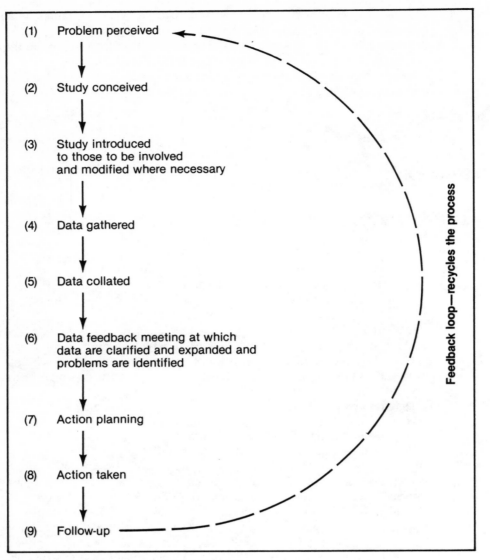

(1)   Problem perceived

(2)   Study conceived

(3)   Study introduced
      to those to be involved
      and modified where necessary

(4)   Data gathered

(5)   Data collated

(6)   Data feedback meeting at which
      data are clarified and expanded and
      problems are identified

(7)   Action planning

(8)   Action taken

(9)   Follow-up

Feedback loop—recycles the process

Reproduced by permission of the author, John J. Sherwood.

Figure 3. Action Research Model

Assessing Internal HRD Needs and Organizational Readiness

Let us assume that as a key decision maker you decide to explore the feasibility of developing a shared service. Generally, you will do some internal planning before you contact other institutions. You will need to answer the following four quesions:

- What are the HRD needs of your institution?
- What is your HRD investment?
- How effective is your existing HRD system?
- What is the HRD posture of your CEO?

Assessing HRD Needs

The components of an HRD system include management and supervisory development, assessment training, nursing education, orientation processes, upward mobility and career development training, nonnursing staff development, professional development for HRD staff, physician and trustee education, community and patient education, and other opportunities. In figure 4, page 22, a sample instrument developed for a hypothetical hospital is presented. The circles represent the response of Hospital A to the question, "What are your HRD needs?"

Hospital A ranked the degree to which each need was being met and how important that need was. This simple diagnosis of the HRD needs of Hospital A yields the following observations:

- Most needs are fairly well met and of low priority (for example, on-the-job training for support personnel). Thus, one can assume that these needs are not critical enough to warrant serious attention.
- A few needs (such as medical secretary training) are well met, indicating a real strength, one that other hospitals could tap if a shared service were developed.
- Many needs are poorly met and are viewed as having a high priority (such as executive education, middle manager development, and patient education).

This simple assessment, then, tells Hospital A that it has some critical, unmet HRD needs that a shared service, under the right circumstances, could support.

Determining HRD Investment

A second question concerns a facility's HRD investment. In response to a brief self-test[2] (see figure 5, page 24), Hospital A indicated that it was not clear on the costs—direct and indirect—of its present involvement in HRD. Essential to making a decision about whether to enter a shared service arrangement is a knowledge of present investment in HRD activities and the impact that involvement in a multihospital arrangement could have on the level or return on the investment. This self-test, designed by the Maryland Hospital Education Institute in collaboration with the American Hospital Association, is backed up by a more extensive manual describing how to conduct a full human resources development audit.[3] If you're not sure of the answers to these questions, your organization probably could benefit from an audit of its human resource development activities (see appendix A).

Done systematically, you should be able to audit these areas:
- The extent to which certain HRD activities are justified
- Deficiencies in the delivery of HRD services
- The costs, direct and indirect, of facility-sponsored programs
- The costs for similar off-site programs
- The percentage of investment allocated to various personnel groups in the institution

Hospitals that have completed this detailed audit generally reported that they were startled by how inattentive they had been to the level and quality of the investment made in HRD activities. One hospital, for example, discovered that its real HRD investment exceeded $1,000,000, and worse, that no one was clearly responsible for managing that investment. Needless to say, that hospital began to manage its HRD activities more carefully to ensure that its return on investment could justify the expenditure and support long-range objectives.

Assessing the Effectiveness of the Present System

The third question is: How effective is your present HRD system? Though the HRD audit provides some data in this area, more is generally needed. Hospital A assessed its HRD function by completing the self-test that appears in figure 6, page 25.[4] Hospital A's profile would be fairly typical of most hospital-based HRD functions. If we examine the data, we can identify these patterns:

- Hospital A does not have a good handle on assessment of needs or the performance of the HRD functions (questions 8-11).
- The HRD function is seen as taking into account the present state of needs (question 1).

Instructions: Listed below are various HRD needs that may affect job performance and satisfaction. For each item listed, indicate the extent to which your hospital meets each HRD need and how important improvement in that area is.

HRD Need	To What Extent Are HRD Needs Being Met? (circle one)					How Important Is Improvement? (circle one)			
	Totally Met	Well Met	Fairly Well Met	Poorly Met	Not Met at All	Critical	High Priority	Low Priority	No Change Needed
Management and supervisory development									
Executive education	1	2	3	(4)	5	4	(3)	2	1
Middle-manager development	1	2	3	(4)	5	4	(3)	2	1
First-line supervisory development	1	2	(3)	4	5	4	3	(2)	1
Assessment training									
Presupervisory assessment program	1	2	(3)	4	5	4	3	(2)	1
Nursing education									
Clinical skills training	1	2	(3)	4	5	4	(3)	2	1
New product usage	1	2	(3)	4	5	4	3	(2)	1
Interpersonal skills development	1	2	(3)	4	5	4	(3)	2	1
Degree programs	1	2	(3)	4	5	4	3	(2)	1
Orientation processes									
New employee training	1	2	(3)	4	5	4	(3)	2	1
New graduate internship	1	2	(3)	4	5	4	3	(2)	1
RN refresher training	1	2	3	(4)	5	4	3	(2)	1
Upward mobility training									
Clerical/secretarial training	1	(2)	3	4	5	4	(3)	2	1
GED high school equivalency	1	(2)	3	4	5	4	3	(2)	1
Medical secretary training	1	(2)	3	4	5	4	3	(2)	1
Career ladder training	1	2	3	(4)	5	4	3	(2)	1

Career development training

Item										
Career counseling	1	2	3	4	5	1	2	(3)	(4)	5
Career planning	1	2	3	4	5	1	(2)	3	(4)	5
Educational and occupational referral	1	2	(3)	4	5	1	(2)	3	(4)	5
Tuition assistance	1	2	3	4	5	1	(2)	3	4	5

Nonnursing staff development and training

Item										
On-the-job training for support personnel (such as housekeeping)	1	2	(3)	4	5	1	(2)	3	4	5
Technical training for ancillary service workers (such as clinical labs)	1	2	(3)	4	5	1	2	(3)	4	5

Professional development for HRD staff

Item										
Training for trainers	1	2	3	(4)	5	1	2	(3)	4	5
Consulting skills	1	2	3	(4)	5	1	(2)	3	4	5
Organizational development	1	2	3	4	(5)	1	(2)	3	4	5

Item										
Physician education	1	2	3	(4)	5	1	2	(3)	4	5
Trustee education	1	2	3	(4)	5	1	2	(3)	4	5

Community and patient education

Item										
Patient education	1	2	3	4	5	1	2	3	(4)	5
Community education	1	2	3	4	5	1	2	(3)	(4)	5

Other (fill in)

Item										
Audiovisual resources	1	2	(3)	4	5	1	2	(3)	4	5
Affirmative action plans	1	2	3	4	5	1	2	(3)	4	5
	1	2	3	4	5	1	2	3	4	5

Figure 4. Instrument to Assess HRD Needs

Question	Do You Know? (circle one)	
	Yes	Not Sure
1. What percentage of the institution's budget is invested in education and training?	Y	(NS)
2. Which of the following groups receives the greatest (and the least) amount of training: top administration, nurses, medical staff, housekeeping, maintenance, social service, physical therapy, other?	(Y)	NS
3. How much does the institution expend on tuition, books, education-related travel, and paid time off for participants?	Y	(NS)
4. How much of the HRD investment is spent on internal versus outside educational programs?	Y	(NS)
5. How much of the HRD investment is spent on a formal continuing education program as opposed to trade association and singular meetings?	Y	(NS)
6. What proportion of the HRD investment goes for technical training? For training to prepare employees for promotion? For maintaining employees' professional standing? For fringe benefits?	Y	(NS)
7. How effectively are training programs achieving their objective, in terms of supervisors' perceptions of employees' posttraining performance?	Y	(NS)

Reprinted with the permission of the Maryland Hospital Education Institute.

Figure 5. Self-Test to Determine HRD Investment

- The hospital tends to conduct activities that are not well targeted to specific change objectives.
- It enjoys the tentative support of key actors in the system

One might conclude that involvement in a shared HRD service could provide Hospital A with the resources and expertise to strengthen its internal system as well as deliver services to its employees. Some shared services invest significant resources in developing HRD professionals to improve their internal systems.

Assessing the CEO's HRD Posture

The final question needing an answer in step 1 is: what is the HRD posture of your CEO? In chapter 1, you examined this issue. The CEO of Hospital A probably would have responded yes to 12 questions, indicating that although he views HRD as more than a luxury, he does not view it as critical to the attainment of the institution's goals. The point here is that the support of the CEO can be attained if the potential benefits of HRD activity, whether in a shared service or under some other arrangement, are made clear to him.

The data you have collected in step 1 are adequate to help you decide whether to proceed with your planning. However, you must keep in mind the future need to do

Question	Does the HRD Function: (circle one)		
	Yes	No	Sometimes
1. Take into account the present state of needs of individuals, groups, and the organization?	(Y)	N	S
2. Include activities based upon clear and measurable objectives so that progress can be measured?	Y	N	(S)
3. Contain activities based on some criteria for successful growth, learning, and performance of individuals?	Y	N	(S)
4. Meet the unique needs of the hospital?	Y	N	(S)
5. Meet the ongoing and changing needs of the institution?	Y	N	(S)
6. Stress skill development for actual behavioral or performance competency?	Y	N	(S)
7. Employ professionals who are prepared by education, practice, skill, and ethics to manage the functions assigned to them?	Y	N	(S)
8. Operate with a clearly articulated value system in which its purposes are clear and philosophically consistent with the norms, values, expectations, and goals of the hospital?	Y	(N)	S
9. Contain activities based on realistic assessments of the future needs of the organization and individuals within it?	Y	(N)	S
10. Contain a meaningful process for assessing its performance and impact?	Y	(N)	S
11. Operate on a solid information base so that data can be stored, retrieved, and updated to serve the organization and provide planning based on previous experience?	Y	(N)	S
12. Have the interest, involvement, commitment, and support of the administrator, top management, and informal leaders in the system?	Y	N	(S)
13. Strengthen the hospital's desire and ability to cope with the problems facing it and to change with a high degree of commitment?	Y	N	(S)
14. Operate within an organizational structure that facilitates rather than blocks performance and impact?	Y	N	(S)

Adapted and reprinted with the permission of Organization Renewal, Inc., Bethesda, MD.

Figure 6. Self-Test to Assess Performance and Impact of HRD Function

more specific analysis for whatever program areas you move into as you plan steps 8 and 12. For example, if you do agree to form a shared HRD service to deal with management education, you may choose to use an instrument like the assessment tool displayed in appendix A. Appendix B presents an example of a survey tool used by the Manchester Health Education Consortium. Our task here is not to provide you with a detailed discussion of diagnostic tools, but to make you aware of the need for other sources and refer you to them.

Environmental Readiness

If you have completed step 1, you may have decided that a shared HRD service can help you meet your internal HRD needs. But such an arrangement is feasible only if the right conditions exist in the larger system of which you are a part. Two questions must be answered:

- Is the environment ready for the development of a shared service?
- What barriers might you face and what is the likelihood that you can overcome them?

Few attempts to establish multihospital efforts fail because needs cannot be identified and acted upon; they fail because forces in the environment block attempts. An important task, then, is to identify those barriers and develop strategies to minimize their negative effects.

Hospital A continued its planning in step 2 by assessing its view of environmental readiness of the system by completing the self-test shown in figure 7, opposite.[5]

By examining this particular profile, one can draw several conclusions:

- Hospital A is particularly concerned about the historical alignment of institutions (because two community hospitals have been in a five-year struggle with the HSA over expansion plans), the time factor involved in developing a shared service, and the HRD posture of several CEOs in the area. With the exception of the historical alignment issue, however, it believes it is quite likely the other two barriers can be overcome.
- Many issues, such as the fear of bigness (in this case, sharing services with a large medical center with expansion plans) and certain personality conflicts are of some concern and may be difficult to change.
- Other factors, such as the ability to reach contractual agreements, are not problematic and could serve to facilitate the development of shared service agreement.

These issues are real and difficult. However, awareness of their force and adequate planning can prevent them from becoming stumbling blocks. (Participants at a national research conference identified many barriers they had experienced and developed a list of strategies they had used to overcome them, see table 2, pages 29-31.) A joint effort to build a shared service in a limited area such as HRD often results in an improvement in relations between and among institutions. Thus, the shared service becomes a vehicle for exploring options in other areas.

Initiating Contact with Other Institutions

If you have an assessment of need and a sense of the barriers you may face, and if the signs are promising, you may choose to initiate informal discussions with key people from other institutions. It is important that you develop a careful strategy. You must identify institutions that are ready to explore a shared service, determine why they are ready and what the implications may be for you if they respond positively. You can also single out those areas that may require particular attention in any subsequent discussions.

Instructions: Listed below are factors that could concern persons involved in developing a shared service. Read each and indicate (1) how concerned you would be about that factor if you were considering a shared service and (2) how likely you think it is that you can overcome the barrier.

Areas of Potential Concern	How Concerned Are You? (circle one)					Will This Barrier Be Overcome? (circle one)			
	Significant Concern	Much Concern	Some Concern	Little Concern	No Concern	Very Likely	Quite Likely	Not Very Likely	Not Likely at All
Historical alignment of institutions	1	(2)	3	4	5	4	3	(2)	1
Lack of precedent (will costs increase? decrease?)	1	2	(3)	4	5	4	(3)	2	1
Membership in a cooperative structure that would not be local	1	2	(3)	4	5	4	(3)	2	1
Fear of bigness ("big brother" syndrome)	1	2	(3)	4	5	4	3	(2)	1
Inability to reach clear contractual agreements	1	2	3	(4)	5	4	(3)	2	1
Conviction that autonomy and competition are better than sharing	1	2	(3)	4	5	4	(3)	2	1
Different types of hospitals and ownership	1	2	3	(4)	5	4	(3)	2	1
Personality conflicts	1	2	(3)	4	5	4	3	(2)	1
The time factor involved	1	(2)	3	4	5	4	(3)	2	1

Figure 7. Self-Test to Assess Environmental Readiness for Shared HRD Services (continued on next page)

Instructions: *Listed below are factors that could concern persons involved in developing a shared service. Read each and indicate (1) how concerned you would be about that factor if you were considering a shared service and (2) how likely you think it is that you can overcome the barrier.*

Areas of Potential Concern	How Concerned Are You? (circle one)					Will This Barrier Be Overcome? (circle one)			
	Significant Concern	Much Concern	Some Concern	Little Concern	No Concern	Very Likely	Quite Likely	Not Very Likely	Not Likely at All
Compromising the control and identity of an institution	1	2	(3)	4	5	4	(3)	2	1
Geographical distance between hospitals	1	2	(3)	4	5	4	3	(2)	1
Philosophical differences	1	2	(3)	4	5	4	(3)	2	1
Vested interests	1	2	(3)	4	5	4	(3)	2	1
Community pride	1	2	3	(4)	5	4	(3)	2	1
HRD posture of other CEOs	1	(2)	3	4	5	4	(3)	2	1
Fit between/among HRD needs of potential institutions	1	2	(3)	4	5	4	(3)	2	1
Organizational readiness of other institutions	1	2	(3)	4	5	4	3	(2)	1

Figure 7. Self-Test to Assess Environmental Readiness for Shared HRD Services (continued)

Table 2. Strategies for Implementation Problems

Problem	Successful Strategies
Funding (finding the money, time, and other resources needed to produce needed programs)	1. A well-organized planning process that provides accurate data about costs, services rendered, return on investment 2. Involve the administrators of the member agencies in the decision-making process 3. Address the needs of the "funding agencies" 4. Establish priorities for needs and invest energies in areas that provide the most payoff to the funding agencies 5. Write grants for "start up" money and for projects such as patient education, health education, emergency medical services 6. Develop a marketing system for programs developed that might make money for you
Development of a cooperative working relationship between agencies that have traditionally not worked together cooperatively	1. Create decision-making groups with representation of the agencies involved, giving them control over the direction of the effort 2. Develop a system that can assess the needs of each institution (include present education activities, education resources) 3. Provide opportunities for individual organizations to get their share of visibility 4. Start with small efforts in order to realize success and move slowly to more complex areas
Development of legitimacy and credibility	1. Start where there is the greatest probability of success 2. Be very clear about who you are, what you can and cannot do; don't create unrealistic expectations. 3. Be patient; don't expect people to be on board the first day 4. Don't promise more than you can deliver
Competition with other regional education providers, such as hospital associations and education organizations	1. Keep your emphasis on grass-roots planning to meet local needs 2. Explore possibilities of cosponsoring programs with other regional education providers when appropriate 3. Recognize that some programs can be developed and offered more effectively by others 4. Try to keep the issues regarding competition on the table so they can be discussed openly; competition can be a positive force, and only unnecessary duplication should be a concern
Development of organizational support (administration, middle managers, and staff)	(A continuing theme in this book)
Large geographical territory	1. Develop regional programs 2. Encourage several member agencies to do some joint programming in their local area

(continued on next page)

Table 2. Strategies for Implementation Problems (continued)

Problem	Successful Strategies
Sharing of education software	1. Develop an audiovisual resource catalog 2. Standardize various pieces of audiovisual equipment
Lack of solid internal education systems in member agencies	1. Encourage the development of a task force within the institution to facilitate the development of institutionwide and agencywide education 2. Maintain contact with the administrator and give him constant feedback about the process; don't be afraid to make recommendations when appropriate. 3. Provide training for the education staff 4. Provide training for department heads regarding the development of their employees
Overextension (trying to do too much with the limited resources available)	1. Develop clear and measurable objectives each year that are approved by the decision-making body 2. Say "no" 3. Get in touch with what you are trying to prove, to whom, and why
Development of broad-based organizational and community support	1. Involve a broad section of all appropriate groups in the decision-making process, ask for their advice and input, or simply keep them informed 2. Whenever possible, encourage coordination and cooperation with community agencies 3. Demonstrate a strong commitment to sharing in your behavior, not just your words 4. Make use of public media such as newspapers, radio, institutional newsletters
Project evaluation	1. Have clear and measurable organizational objectives to provide a baseline for project evaluation 2. Design an evaluation system that attempts to get data on actual change in performance on the job 3. Make use of external evaluators on occasion 4. Provide training for agency education staff relating to evaluation
Amount of time required to make a shared education service work	1. Demonstrate concern for people's time by running effective and efficient meetings, involving people at the appropriate levels of decision making, and so forth 2. Offer help and plan programs to reduce some of the energy drain 3. Reinforce the importance of the participation of others in the process and keep a focus on the successes that result from such efforts

Table 2. Strategies for Implementation Problems (continued)

Problem	Successful Strategies
Organizational competition	1. Bring people together on all levels, and get them talking to one another 2. Recognize the usefulness of competition and provide for visibility of individual agencies when appropriate 3. Encourage the development and offering of multiagency programs 4. Document the payoffs resulting from sharing, and constantly explore the possibilities for increased sharing
Poor use of consortium services by some members	1. Keep the administrator and education department aware of the situation 2. Analyze the problem areas on an ongoing basis 3. Restructure the delivery system when indicated

Initiating Discussions

Once a positive decision has been reached about initiating contact with other institutions in the area, discussions with key leaders can begin. Then, leaders in these institutions must appraise their internal HRD needs and organizational readiness (that is, complete step 1) and determine environmental readiness (step 2). You may choose to share the results of your diagnostic process with them as a way of opening more dialog.

Initiating Exploratory Planning

A decision point to initiate exploratory planning is self-explanatory. Each institution needs to commit itself to the tasks of the second stage; the outcome of that stage will be an agreement to organize or a decision not to proceed. As we review the sequence of the preaffiliation stage, we realize that there are many ways to walk the same path. For example, a group of hospitals could move directly to establish a joint study group to accomplish steps 1 through 6 simultaneously. In fact, some shared services began by hiring a consultant or full-time staff to do the same tasks. What is important is to avoid premature steps that may lead to disappointment or difficulty.

Successfully negotiating the preaffiliation stage requires a particular set of leadership skills. During this phase, the most critical leadership quality required is political sensitivity, that is, the ability to deal competently and discretely with various constituencies. Each potential member brings to the effort a unique set of needs. Many of the hospitals, especially those located in proximity to one another, may have a history of competing with one another, and, more than likely, each key actor will have a unique style and personality. Developing common ground and a serious commitment to a multi-institutional effort demands careful orchestrating.

The second quality needed is the ability to demonstrate competence and to communicate confidence that something worthwhile can come from a cooperative effort. There is natural resistance to cooperative efforts, and the leaders at this stage have to be able to instill confidence and trust that they know what they are doing and where they are going.

The third necessary quality is that of organizational sensitivity. Change in any part of a system is going to result in additional changes in other systems or subunits. Key leaders must have a sensitivity to potential barriers, pockets of resistance, or problems that might develop. They also must be capable of developing strategies to address those problems.

NOTES

1. Developed by John Sherwood and presented at a seminar sponsored by the NTL Institute.

2. A questionnaire developed for marketing *Guidelines and Procedures for Measuring Accountability in Human Resource Development*. Baltimore: ASHET, Maryland Chapter, 1976.

3. American Society for Health Manpower, Education, and Training, Maryland Chapter. *Guidelines and Procedures for Measuring Accountability in Human Resource Development*. Baltimore: ASHET, Maryland Chapter, 1976.

4. Nippit, G. *Human Resource Development Assessment Inventory*. Bethesda, MD: Organization Renewal, Inc., 1976.

5. Adapted by the authors from DesRoches, H. B. Breaking down barriers to shared services. *Trustee,* August 1977, pp. 34-36.

Chapter 4

The Formation Stage

Negotiating the formation stage requires imagination, strategic planning, and the careful involvement of key decision makers. The most creative work occurs during this phase and, if successfully completed, can lead to an agreement to organize a shared HRD service. Thus, a vision is transformed into reality. You will know who will join, whether you will become a member, and what you want to get done.

Organizing the Internal Decision-Making Group

When attempting to organize the internal decision-making group of a shared service, three questions must be answered:

- Who should assume internal leadership to plan the shared service and to coordinate it once developed?
- Who should be involved in the group and how should their tasks be defined?
- How should you, as a leader, approach the group?

The leadership must come from the top if you want to build an organization that can meet critical needs. The principles of planned change outlined in chapter 2 need to be considered each step of the way. Too often, one of three scenarios is played out: the task is delegated to HRD staff people, everyone is involved in the process, or one or two people hold all the information or power and go it alone. Each scenario is deadly. The first lessens the importance of the process, the second complicates it, and the third precludes building the necessary support. The ideal is to build a group composed of creative, flexible people, with position power, expert power, and creative power fully represented.

The reality is that there are probably as many reasons, conscious and unconscious, rational and irrational, for not participating in a shared service as there are for participating. It is important, therefore, to keep the issue of "organizational support" in mind at all times as one is going through the implementation phase. The support of administrators, senior managers, department heads, and HRD people will vary greatly from institution to institution. Competition as a way of controlling hospital costs is gaining in popularity. Increasing competition makes successful collaborative efforts significantly more difficult but not impossible. The support of significant managers within the hospital will be affected by the level of competition among member hospitals, turf issues within institutions, varying priorities, interpersonal relations, historical developments, and so on.

Motives for Involvement

Although substantial evidence suggests that HRD services can be developed and

33

delivered in a cost effective manner, a whole range of motives for engaging in such efforts usually exists and has a significant impact on the success or failure of shared service efforts. There are three main categories of motives: rational, political, and normative (that is, based on beliefs and values).[1]

The rational motives for participating in shared services are probably the most obvious and, at least on the surface, the most common reasons given for participation. They include payoffs such as reduced HRD costs, more efficient use of resources, reduction of duplication, an increase in the sophistication of programs, and so on. It is not difficult to demonstrate that a well-managed shared service can provide all of the above payoffs. Thus, it seems logical to move ahead.

The political motives are far more complex and difficult to assess. There are a significant number of political issues to be considered in a shared service that can result in either support or resistance. These issues exist on both a broad organizational and individual level. They include such factors as the image created in the community; the evidence or cooperation for health systems planning; the prestige of accomplishment in areas not tackled by others; the visibility that a hospital might attain on a regional level; the opportunity for individual hospitals and their staffs to demonstrate expertise; the strengthening of individual and organizational relationships; the belief that HRD is a relatively "safe" area in which to build cooperative ventures; the degree to which the service is in competition with the services of key individuals within member organizations, colleges, universities, or associations; and the degree of conflict among key people or organizations.

The normative motives have more to do with people's belief systems, that is, what they value, believe in, have as priorities, or care about. The degree to which people at various levels of the system are committed to human resource development activities in general or to specific aspects of it (such as management development or community health education) will have a significant impact on the level of support present.

Seldom is there any one primary motivating factor in a shared HRD service. There are as many mixtures of motivation as there are people and organizations involved in the process. It is also realistic to assume that motives will change as the process develops and as persons discover what a shared HRD service can and cannot do for them. The task is to keep in tune with those motivations as much as possible in order to continue developing strategies for developing support. A primary principle for developing support in any organizational change or development effort is to involve key people in an appropriate manner. The primary actors that you need to be concerned about are administrators, senior managers, department heads, first-line managers, educators, and staff.

Administrative Support

The support of the administrators of participating institutions, especially during the initial stages of the effort, is absolutely essential. Too often, the responsibility for making shared services work is delegated to lower level managers who do not have decision-making power and who have no control over many of the significant barriers that may be expected. If the administrator is not directly involved in the process, or if a senior manager with decision-making responsibility has not been delegated the task, serious questions should be raised as to whether or not sufficient support exists to move ahead.

Key indicators that should be examined in assessing administrative support are the time that the CEO is willing to commit to the effort; the willingness of the CEO to commit hard money to the effort; and the degree to which the CEO provides access to himself, key people, information, and resources within his organization. Whatever structures are going to be set up to manage and develop the effort, a process should be designed at the start to keep the administrator engaged in the process. This can be accomplished through their inclusion in the internal decision-making group or the governance structure, through periodic meetings with the professional staff, through occasional attendance at senior administrative meetings, or through informal communication (such as telephone updates and breakfast meetings) and written reports.

Senior Manager Support

The next level of administration is frequently the most difficult to engage in the process. Senior managers generally do not have direct contact with the results of programming. This factor causes many of them to be defensive when asked for input because they frequently do not have any firsthand data. They are very much caught in the middle between the administrator's expectations regarding the long-term development of the hospital and the day-to-day crises experienced by those who report to them. The last thing that they need is a new project that could be perceived as increasing their work load and perhaps exposing some of their weaknesses.

Although their participation and support during the initial stages of the effort may not appear critical, they will have a significant impact on the continued funding of the project. If participation in the project is forced upon them by the administrator, there will be an uphill battle throughout the development of the effort.

Therefore, they need to be involved, whenever possible, in the task force making the initial decisions, asked for input individually regarding participation in the program and the types of services that might be provided, and kept informed, both formally and informally, about the project's development and problems. Developing support at this level will result in a greater availability of key department heads and a more consistent emphasis on the importance of human resource development efforts. These two elements are among the cornerstones for success.

A word of caution: As indicated above, a common practice is to assign HRD responsibilities to a midlevel staff person. Although this may be appropriate in light of that person's role and responsibilities, it is fraught with dangers because that person does not have substantial line authority. There is no question that this person should be involved in the process in a significant way; however, if the person is going to have primary responsibility, it is critical that he or she have the necessary authority as well.

At the minimum, the senior administrative team should keep the process of the internal group on its regular agenda. The team also should be included in any decisions regarding services to be delivered within its institution, involved in problem solving regarding issues that affect it, and receive ongoing evaluation data.

Department Head and First-Line Supervisor Support

The department heads and first-line supervisors possess a wealth of data concerning the learning needs of staff. They also know the various aspects of the organization that function as barriers to employee development. Because of the numerous disciplines involved in hospitals, it is not possible for any staff person to meet all of the needs involved. Middle and first-line managers are therefore the primary sources of such expertise. They are able to provide data for targeting the programs to more effectively meet the needs of their staff. They frequently have the expertise to serve as faulty for specific programs, and they are aware of other resources in the area that might be helpful.

Because the primary responsibility for developing the line staff falls on the shoulders of middle and first-line managers, a successful shared service can be very helpful to them in meeting this responsibility. Potentially, they are the greatest supporters of the services provided. On the other hand, if they are not part of the effort, they can effectively block the participation of their staff. They should be involved heavily in the needs assessment process and the planning of specific programs, and they should be invited to serve as faculty when appropriate. Informal relationships with them should be developed.

Educator and Staff Support

The internal HRD functions in hospitals across the country are rapidly growing in size and sophistication, ranging from hospitalwide education systems to intensive human resource development efforts. Depending upon how a shared HRD effort is managed, it will be seen as either a support for the development of the internal education system or a competitor. The reality is that the two groups are about the same business and could be competing for the same resources. The internal department and the shared service should be integrated carefully, with a clear definition and understanding of the role and function of each group.

The key to this relationship is to develop a sound working relationship so that both sides experience the support of the other and value the input and expertise that the other can provide. Ideally, the staff of each group can function as consultants to the other on the development of their systems. Theoretically, the two groups share goals, but it is easy to slip into conflict related to power, turf issues, and so on.

As in any significant change effort, a certain amount of resistance is to be expected, and it is important that you be prepared to develop conscious strategies to overcome this resistance as to attempt to implement your shared service. Thus, it is obvious that representatives from each of these groups need to be involved in the internal decision-making group.

When you made your decision to proceed in step 6, you may have worked with a few key actors, or even formed a full-fledged planning group. If you need to form a new group, keep these pointers in mind:[2]

- Explain why the group is being formed. Provide all the facts about the reason for changing. If there are risks, acknowledge them, but tell why the risks are worthwhile. Show what you have done to minimize the risk.
- Name the benefits that could result from the program/service—Don't exaggerate, but list them objectively. Not to do so would be like a salesperson not telling a customer what the product can do.
- Seek questions and answer them. This will stop rumors that inevitably arise during an organizational change.
- Invite participation. Ask for suggestions, because the people involved know the situation best. Changes work out most favorably when those concerned have a part in suggesting the change.
- Avoid surprise. Surprise stirs unreasoning opposition more than any other factor because those involved don't have time to think. Their emotions take over, and such emotions are likely to be negative.
- Acknowledge the rough spots. In selling an organizational change, we tend to make it sound simple, presenting a clear-cut chart and neat lines of responsibilities. But even a minor change is rarely simple. Admit it, and tell how you plan to smooth the shift.
- Set standards. Give a date when you want the change to be completed. Tell what you want it to accomplish. What are the penalities for failure? The rewards for success?
- Contact informal leaders. Let them know what is going on in particular detail.
- Praise performance. People in any new situation are anxious, and positive reinforcement helps.
- Repeat important points. To get across something complex, you must tell the story over and over, using fresh examples and different approaches.

Matching Needs and Readiness Levels

Step 8 in the formation stage consists of matching needs and readiness levels in an effort to identify joint goals and missions. During this step, you are seeking answers to four basic questions:

- Is there a fit between needs and readiness levels?
- If the fit is not clear, are there areas for potential action?
- How would you summarize the basic mission of a shared service venture?
- Can you identify goals for cooperative action?

During the preaffiliation phase, you succeeded in bringing about enough agreement to initiate exploratory planning at an interinstitutional level. Assuming that the fit between needs, readiness levels, and targets for change is in place, you should now seek an agreement to form an organization. You face the task of developing an organizational form that will enable you to carry out those functions you consider most important.

The first question you must ask is, "Do we have a fit?" No simple answer will emerge in at least in 90 percent of the situations you may face. A second question is, "How ready are we for each activity?" You may find, for example, that different organizations have different readiness levels for different needs. All organizations may express a need for management development training, yet two organizations may be very ready to begin such efforts and three others may be in no position to start without some preparatory work. A third question is, "Where do we start, and what's really most important?" Resource, political, environmental, and personnel factors will force you to focus your efforts in areas where need and payoff are the highest. Your work in steps 8 and 9 will prepare you to make your final decision to proceed with the development of a shared service in step 10. A critical juncture will come when you reach an agreement to organize.

Identifying Needs That Match

The matching matrix, figure 8, page 38, will help you answer the question: Do we have needs that fit? A hypothetical example will be used to illustrate the use of the matrix. Assume that four hospitals, ranging in bed capacity from 83 to 404, are trying to build a shared service. They completed their initial diagnostic work and agreed that a shared service may help them meet some of their HRD needs. In the matrix, the hospitals are listed along the top and the needs along the side. Then, the need values (determined by adding responses from each side of the scale provided in figure 4, page 22) of each potential program area for each hospital are listed. Hospitals A and B, for example, rank "Middle manager development" at 7.0, meaning that it is a "poorly met" need and has a "high priority." Any figure of 5.5 or higher can be viewed as a blip on the radar screen that needs to be analyzed.

An analysis of the matrix indicates that the needs that appear to be the most critical for the four hospitals *as a group* include:

1. Training for HRD professionals
2. Executive education
3. Middle-manager education
4. Career counseling
5. On-the-job training for support personnel
6. Consulting skills for HRD professionals and others
7. Educational and occupational referral
8. Technical training for ancillary personnel
9. Organizational development
10. Patient education

In general, then, we have a good fit; however, what do we say about Hospital D, whose needs seem less intense and quite different? One possibility is that it would not

Need Area	Hospital				Mean
	A	B	C	D	
Executive education	7	7	8	4	6.5
Middle-manager development	7	7	8	4	6.5
First-line supervisory development	5	6	7	3	5.3
Presupervisory assessment program	5	7	4	5	5.3
Clinical skill training	6	7	5	4	5.5
New product usage	5	5	6	4	5.0
Interpersonal skills development	6	6	5	4	5.3
Degree programs	5	5	5	5	5.0
New employee training	6	7	4	4	5.3
New graduate internship	5	5	4	4	4.5
RN refresher training	6	5	6	4	5.3
Clerical/secretarial training	6	7	5	2	5.0
GED high school equivalency	4	5	6	4	4.8
Medical secretary/training	4	5	3	2	3.5
Career ladder training	6	6	5	5	5.5
Career counseling	7	6	6	5	6.0
Career planning	6	6	4	5	5.3
Educational and occupational referral	6	6	6	5	5.8
Tuition assistance	5	6	5	3	4.8
On-the-job training for support personnel (for example, housekeeping)	5	8	7	4	6.0
Technical training for ancillary service workers (for example, clinical laboratories)	6	7	6	4	5.8
Training for trainers	7	7	7	6	6.8
Consulting skills	6	6	5	7	6.0
Organizational development	7	5	5	6	5.8
Physician education	6	4	4	7	5.3
Trustee education	6	7	5	4	5.5
Patient education	8	7	4	4	5.8
Community education	6	6	5	5	5.5
AV resources	7	-	-	-	7.0
Affirmative action	-	-	-	8	8.0

Figure 8. Matrix for Determining Matching Needs

fare well in this shared service because the most critical needs of the others are those that it has already been able to address. A second possibility is that Hospital D's strength in the high need areas of others, for example, management and supervisory development, could be an asset to the shared service, assuming that other organizations can help it address those areas, such as physician education and affirmative action, where it sees a real need. Thus, Hospital D could, at this point, decide that a shared service would not address its needs, or it could seek to develop an organization that would meet differing needs, in a collaborative fashion. Important at this point is that you find a way to discuss the fits you find in your matrixes.

Reaffirming Readiness

At this point, you know those activities that could be addressed in the hypothetical example above; the hospitals may want to pursue efforts in any or all of the top 10 areas. But how ready is each institution to pursue this course, to enter into a shared service agreement that carries expectations and commitments? In steps 1 and 2, you examined this question, assessing the readiness level of your own institution and the readiness of others in the environment.

You, and other institutions, agreed to proceed in steps 3 and 6. Now the readiness level of each institution needs to be discussed in a more formal way by examining data developed in earlier steps. At this point, chances are good that you have an adequate fit and can proceed with identifying a mission and goals.

Ranking Needs

Having a ranking of needs derived from the original questionnaires you could use this raw data and agree to the list of top 10 needs. But further analysis can clarify thinking further. Using a decision-making matrix (see figure 9, page 40),[3] you can compare each need against every other need systematically, thus giving yourself a truer picture of actual priorities. Using this tool, a new list of priorities emerges. In order of desending importance, they are:

1. Patient education
2. Clinical skills training
3. Middle manager development
4. Executive education
5. Trustee education
6. Community education
7. On-the-job training—support personnel
8. Technical training—ancillary personnel
9. Training—HRD professionals
10. Consulting skills
11. Organizational development
12. Career ladder training
13. Career counseling
14. Educational and occupational referral

Note, for example, that patient education moves from number 10 to number 1 after a better sorting process. These needs, then, are those viewed as most important. Now you can begin more formal planning.

You have now found a fit (or else have aborted the effort), have decided how ready you are for specific activities and developed realistic expectations, and have decided where to start and what's most important. In short, you have roughly defined your basic raison d'etre.

Drafting a Mission and Goals Statement

Identifying a mission and goals statement is the subject of numerous texts and articles, so little time will be spent on the "how to" aspects of the step. The Maryland Hospital Education Institute example (figure 10, page 41) is a fine model.[4] It is a concise, thoughtfully developed statement that focuses the resources and energy of that organization on specific areas. Although a full analysis would require pages, we can highlight some salient features. For example, MHEI:

- Attaches a high priority to applied research and development
- Views itself as a forum, as well as a service organization, for its members
- Concentrates on management, professional, and governance levels in four key result areas
- Clearly defines four objectives, including the development of a new organizational strategy

If you were to diagnose the MHEI system using some of the tools discussed in chapter 2, you would find that this shared service organization is competently run and makes a measurable impact on its members. What is stated in the MHEI document is critical. However, equally important is the MHEI has chosen not to include certain mission

Instructions:
1. List each project twice—once on horizontal line, again on corresponding vertical line.
2. Evaluate no. 1 against no. 2. If *more important,* place X in box under no. 2; if *less important,* leave blank. Repeat with *each* remaining number. Continue to next line; repeat.
3. *Total Xs across* for each number—enter in HORIZONTAL box at bottom; *total spaces down* for each number—enter in VERTICAL box at bottom; *add both* for TOTAL.
4. *Largest* number under TOTAL will be 1 in RANK ORDER; next largest will be 2, and so on. If two or more alternatives have same TOTAL, RANK ORDER is determined by comparing each subjectively against others. (This will not happen unless there is an inconsistency.)

	1 Training HRD professionals	2 Executive education	3 Middle-management education	4 Career counseling	5 On-the-job training—support	6 Consulting skills	7 Educational and occupational referral	8 Technical training—ancillary	9 Organizational development	10 Patient education	11 Clinical skills training	12 Career ladder training	13 Trustee education	14 Community education	Total Xs
1 Training HRD professionals				X		X	X		X			X			5
2 Executive education				X	X	X	X		X			X	X	X	8
3 Middle-management education				X	X	X	X	X	X			X	X	X	9
4 Career counseling						X									1
5 On-the-job training—support						X	X		X			X			4
6 Consulting skills							X		X			X			3
7 Educational and occupational referral												X			1
8 Technical training—ancillary									X						1
9 Organizational development												X			1
10 Patient education											X	X	X	X	4
11 Clinical skills training												X	X	X	3
12 Career ladder training															0
13 Trustee education														X	1
14 Community education															0
Vertical (spaces)	0	1	2	0	2	2	0	5	2	9	9	2	8	8	
Horizontal (Xs)	5	8	9	1	4	3	1	1	1	4	3	0	1	0	
Total	5	9	11	1	6	5	1	6	3	13	12	2	9	8	
Rank Order	9	4	3	13	7	9	13	7	11	1	2	12	4	6	

Figure 9. Matrix for Decision Making

MHEI Mission

The mission of the Maryland Hospital Education Institute is to improve the performance of hospitals and related health care institutions through continuing education, consultation, and applied research and development.

The institute serves its member institutions through its programming and leadership in a forum for communication, with opportunities for education, cooperation, and unification of purpose.

MHEI concentrates on serving people at the management, professional, and governance levels in hospitals and draws direction and resources from them.

MHEI key result areas (program area concentrations)
- Planning and policy (the hospital's response to regulation and other external forces)
- Management development
- Quality assurance and patient safety
- Delivery of care

MHEI Institute Objectives

1. Retain 32 hospitals with a stake in MHEI programming. (A stake is defined as one or more of the following: in-hospital utilization of consultative services; training programs or surveys; the use of more than 100 person-days of training; hospital team attendance at the medical staff conference; involvement of hospital leadership on MHEI board or in key MHEI activities.)

   Recruit 3 new hospital members while retaining at least 50 current members.

2. Deliver at least 3,000 person-days of training in four program area concentrations (clusters); planning and policy/response to regulation, management development, quality assurance, and delivery of care.

   Develop more effective linkages among educational programs, consulting services, and publications within clusters.

   Increase income so that net income from training covers one-third of MHEI's fixed expenses.

3. Deliver contracted-for services carried over from one year to the next, including: building a human resource development system in a new multihospital system, testing new patient education materials, completion of ambulatory care book, production and marketing of a trustee manual, and additional trustee development services for Maryland hospitals.

4. Develop a new organizational strategy and capacity to deliver research and development services and contribute new systems knowledge to the hospital field. These will include: completing multiyear objectives, proposed programs, and a marketing plan; continuing to plan with such national health care organizations as the American College of Surgeons, the American Hospital Association, and the Joint Commission on Accreditation of Hospitals as the prime resources for collaborative effort; receiving contracts or grants for new R&D initiatives.

Reprinted, with permission, from 1979 Annual Report *of the Maryland Hospital Education Institute.*

Figure 10: Example of Mission and Goal Statement

elements or objectives. Some shared services, for example, may choose to focus on nonprofessional HRD needs and view applied research and development as unimportant. What is important is that the final result be sharply focused and accepted by potential members of the shared service.

The next task is to develop a set of goals for the shared service. The goals should be comprehensive and written in such a manner as to describe in concrete, measurable terms exactly what is going to be accomplished (key results) within a specific time period. Although the specific content of an organization's written goals will vary, the following items might be described in some fashion:

- Number of full-time and part-time members
- Total operating budget
- Amount of money to be generated through various sources (membership assessment, contracts, program income, grants, and so forth)
- Assessments to be conducted
- Planning groups to be established
- Training activities (programs, training hours, number of participants to be reached, percentage of population, and so forth)
- Consultation activities
- Marketing activities
- Evaluation activities
- Types of documentation to be maintained

Goals for the total shared service as well as for activities within individual member institutions should be developed in such a manner as to clearly describe where the total resources—manpower, equipment, supplies, and so forth—are being invested. To the degree possible, they also should identify the concrete results that can be expected. For an ongoing shared service, goals should describe normal work activities, improvement activities, and new activities or services.

Well-developed goals:

- Enable the organization to be very clear about where it intends to go and to communicate that to present and potential members
- Provide a baseline for evaluation of the organization on an ongoing and annual basis
- Provide clear bench marks that enable staff to set priorities and decide where to invest its energies
- Provide clear expectations to staff about what it is expected to accomplish and serve as a powerful motivation tool if used effectively

You can refer to a good planning text to help you develop your own mission and goals statements.[5]

When you have completed step 8, you know your function. You are now ready to develop the organizational form and a funding plan, as you start step 9.

Implementing an Organizational Form and Funding Plan

The fact that an organization has a noble and worthy mission is no guarantee that it will succeed. According to various studies of factors involved in the failures of small businesses, roughly 98 percent fail because of managerial weakness; less than 2 percent of the failures are due to factors beyond the control of the persons involved. Those who would attempt to start a shared HRD service might remember that, in the final analysis, a shared service is a business and should be planned and managed like one.

Developing a strong organizational component is a critical element in the development of a successful shared service. The baseline for any successful business effort is the business plan that becomes the road map and guide for success, both programmatically and financially. A well-conceived business plan will help you to:

- Decide on the most appropriate organizational structures
- Choose products and services with a clearer rationale and awareness of expected outcomes and risks
- Set budget guidelines, including a working capital budget and break-even analysis
- Provide a set of financial forecasts based on your rational assumptions about the future
- Monitor your progress and identify problem areas with objective criteria

A publication entitled *Business Planning Guide* is an excellent tool that will help you develop your plan.[6] This publication presents a series of questions that will help you to think out some of the pieces of your business plan. This plan should be in writing and you should use it actively as a tool for the ongoing development of your shared service. You may wish also to use the financial worksheet shown in appendix C.

It may be helpful to walk through major questions to demonstrate a sample business plan for a shared HRD service. Such a model appears at the end of this chapter. Needless to say, the business plan will vary significantly from organization to organization, and it would be a serious mistake simply to copy sections from a model. But such an exercise will demonstrate one approach and help you to understand the process.

The business plan becomes the foundation for the development of your shared service organization. It is a working document that needs to be revised as conditions or the shape or focus of the organization change. Another issue that frequently surfaces is whether we need to incorporate a shared service. Our recommendation is that you use your attorney to help you make such a decision.

Making a Decision

You are now ready to make the final decision. You know what you need, what you expect, what it will cost, the shape of the business plan, and the motives of your potential partners. The compelling questions are: Does a fit exist? Will I realize the return on investment that I expect?

As before, you need to examine the leadership skills required in stage 2, since they differ somewhat from those required in stage 1.

During the formation state, the key leadership skills are diagnosis and negotiation. The foundation for an effective, cooperative effort is a good assessment of the individual and common needs of member institutions. It is critical to manage the negotiation process well so that the priorities of each institution are sufficiently included in the objectives of the project, thus ensuring enthusiasm and commitment to the effort. Long-range and strategic planning skills are also needed during this stage of the process. If the project is to be successful, there must be a clear sense of mission, well-defined objectives, and a set of imaginative but realistic strategies for moving ahead. Finally, the ability to develop a viable organizational structure that will provide an effective and efficient governance system is important. The structure needs to be simple so as not to be overburdening, but adequate enough to involve the right people in the right decisions. Dealing with the governance issue is our next step as we move into stage 3, implementation.

Model Process for Establishing an Organizational Form and Funding Plan for a Shared HRD Service

1. Describe Services

Describe the nature of the shared service briefly, including the types of services, the organizational form (corporation, and so forth), the hours of business, and why it will be successful.

The consortium is a not-for-profit corporation that provides a variety of technical education, management training, and organizational development services to the hospital industry. Its primary market is the hospital industry within Region 1. It will begin its operation on June 1, 1982, and its total operating budget is $130,000. During 1983, services are expected to expand substantially and the total operating budget will amount to $200,000.

The specific services offered by the consortium include:

- Technical education workshops for all allied health personnel working with hospitals (These programs will consist of workshops of one or two days' duration.)
- Core technical programs that will be more substantial technical programs for the purpose of certification or substantial skill development (They will range from 20 to 60 hours in length and will cover coronary care, respiratory care, medical terminology, pharmacology, and nurse's aide training.)
- Senior, middle, and first-line management training programs (More than 150 hours of training programs have been developed and field-tested.)
- Consultation to hospitals regarding human resource development issues as they are related to management development, performance appraisal systems, unionization activities, department head input into budgeting systems, managing mergers, and technical training
- The formal assessment of hospitals for the purpose of identifying their strengths and weaknesses as they attempt to improve their human resource development functions
- Consultation to hospital boards of trustees engaging in self-assessment and development activities
- Consultation to hospital administrators regarding the performance of their senior administrative team

The members of this consortium include hospitals X, Y, Z, and K. The administrators at these four hospitals are committed to the success of the effort, as are a number of key senior managers, personnel directors, and educators.

The consortium will be open on a year-round basis. Its business will be conducted between the hours of 8:30 a.m. and 4:30 p.m.

There will be various models for gaining access to consortium programs:

- Full members will be assessed a membership fee and gain access to all services at no extra charge. Representatives have membership on the board.
- Partial members will have contracts with the project for a combination of services that is clearly defined.
- Individual contracts will be offered for specific pieces of work.
- Centralized programs will be offered and attendance will involve payment of established registration fees.

2. Define the Market

Describe the market that will be served by the organization, including who it is (individuals and organizations), its size, the percentage of the market that is expected, its growth potential, how the organization intends to satisfy the market, and how service(s) will be priced in order to be competitive.

Hospitals today are under a tremendous amount of pressure to meet standards of performance that are higher and more stringent than ever before. The increased activities of government agencies, review organizations, consumer groups, unions, and a host of others accompanied by an increasingly complex medical technology make it clearer than ever that an effective and efficient team of managers and line staff at every level of the modern hospital is critical to its operation and survival. This need is responsible for the rapid development of the relatively new market for services such as those offered by the consortium.

Although most hospitals today are attempting to address the problem of developing their human resources and managers, resources are limited and most efforts tend to be piecemeal, unsystematic, and questionable in their purpose and their expected results. Hospitals that hire external consulting agencies to help them address the problem are frequently frustrated by the fact that the consultant with an industrial or academic background is not truly familiar with the hospital world. It was precisely for this reason that the consortium was founded; namely, to bring the expertise of professional consultants, who have worked closely with the hospital industry, to hospitals that are attempting to improve their human resource development efforts, but in a cooperative and cost-effective manner.

The primary market for the consortium services are four acute-care medical hospitals in Region 1 with a total of 1,500 beds and 5,000 personnel. (The organization has been limited to Region 1 for the immediate future due to the desire to make maximum use of the services and the fact that the consortium's staff resources are quite limited at this time.) There are approximately 10 hospitals of this size in the region, and therefore strong possibility of expansion.

We expect that 90 percent of consortium revenues for 1982 will come from the member hospitals. The additional 10 percent will come from program income from staff of nonmember hospitals who attend centralized programs.

The consortium's data regarding the potential within the primary market described above have been gathered through direct contact with managers from hospitals throughout the region, and contact with professional staff of state and regional hospital associations.

The data confirm that the need for the type of services that the consortium offers is very strong and rapidly increasing due to many of the pressures described earlier.

Consortium staff and associates have had experience with the market described above while working for several competitors described in the following section.

At this point, the strength of the shared service is the experience of the staff and associates delivering management training programs within hospitals. Few other organizations in New England can compete with that experience.

It is also encouraging to note that management training is a significant priority for most hospitals within the region today. With management training as the "foot in the door," consortium staff expects to be 70 percent successful in expanding the initial request for training to include other services.

The consortium expects to attract business from this market in the following manner:

- Referral from member hospitals that have been satisfied with work done in their organizations by consortium staff and associates
- Participation of consortium staff and associates in conferences sponsored by state and regional hospital associations
- Direct contact, through referral, with potential clients
- Selective mailings regarding the general services of the consortium
- Selective packaging and marketing of specific programs and services offered by the shared service

At the present time, the consortium charges $359 for a full day of internal management training, or $450 for a full day of consultation. Clients are charged an additional amount for costs related to room, board, travel, telephone, printed materials, and so forth. These fees are competitive with the fees of other providers in the region who charge from $300 to $700 per day. This fee was computed after developing the enclosed operating budget for 1982 and after surveying the rates of competitors. The present fee schedule covers the operating expenses of the consortium in the following manner:

53% Salaries
12% Fringe benefits
30% Administrative overhead
 5% Profit
100%

3. List Competitors

Describe the competition. Who are your major competitors (internally and externally)? What is the status of their business? Why will you do better than they will? What are the strengths and weaknesses?

Although there is a large number of both for-profit and not-for-profit organizations in the region that offer technical training, management training, and organizational development services, most of them are a significant distance away and offer their services at a very high cost. The tabulation on page 48 lists the primary competitors in the region, accompanied by an assessment of their strengths and weaknesses.

The consortium is competitive with all of the organizations mentioned on the previous page. Present staff members were primary actors in the development of the services offered by organizations A and B, the two primary competitors. The staffs have a broader base of experience in the hospital industry than any of the staff of the competitors mentioned.

This fact is clearly the primary strength of the consortium. On the other hand, its weakest points, at the present time, are that there are still only two full-time staff persons, the funding base is somewhat limited, marketing activities are limited, and the organization has not yet earned a name for itself. All of these factors will change rapidly.

4. Establish Objectives

Describe your organizational objectives, including the services that you intend to offer. What is the range of services? What will the priorities be? How do these services compare with those of others?

We expect to be able to provide approximately 132 days of consultation, 176 days of management training, and 20,000 contract hours of technical training during the first year of operations. The priorities, in order, will be management training programs, consultation, and technical training programs.

The management training programs are of the highest quality and enjoy a strong competitive edge because they are carefully tailored to each institution. The consultation services are also of the highest quality and gain a competitive edge because of the long-term relationship. The technical programs have a competitive edge because they are developed with the help of key managers in the area and are offered locally. All of these services are priced at a level that is significantly lower than those offered by competitors.

5. Determine Space Needs

Describe your need for physical space, including square footage, desirable location, and other special needs such as office, classroom, and meeting space.

The project needs four separate offices, three with approximately 144 square feet each and one with approximately 256 square feet, for a total of 688 square feet. The ideal location would be within a member hospital. If office space is to be rented, it must be at a rate of not more than $7 per square foot.

The project also needs access to classroom space within member institutions and at a centralized space. Classrooms will be used actively on an average of two days per week. If space must be rented, it must cost no more than $50 per day. Meeting space will also be needed but should be able to be provided for without significant difficulties.

6. Perceive Management Needs

Describe the management needs of the organization, including the type of manager (as detailed in a job description, criteria for hiring, salary range, and so forth), types of consultants needed (such as accountant or lawyer), and other staffing needs.

The staffing needs of the project include a full-time director, associate director, coordinator, and a secretary. It also requires approximately three part-time consultants, totaling approximately one-half full-time equivalent.

The director must be a highly skilled project manager with expertise in the areas of program development, fiscal management, staff coaching and supervision, strategic planning, and marketing. He/she must have a high level of organizational, developmental, and consultation skills and a solid background in the development and management of management training activities. Expected salary range is from $30,000 to $35,000.

The associate director must have extensive experience as a management development consultant. The position requires an experienced professional in the areas of program development, consultation, training, and materials development. Expected salary range is from $22,000 to $28,000.

The program coordinator must have a working knowledge of adult education principles, familiarity with hospital-based professionals, good coordination skills, and good writing skills. The position requires a person with good group process skills and strong interpersonal abilities. Expected salary range is from $16,000 to $19,000.

The secretary should be at the level of an executive secretary and have experience in program management, materials development, bookkeeping, and marketing activities. Salary range is from $11,000 to $14,000.

Consultant skills and experience will be dependent on the nature of the work. The fee range will be from $150 to $250 per day.

The project will make limited use of legal and accounting services. The primary need for such services will be for the annual audit.

7. Plan Financial Needs

Describe the financial aspects of the organization, including capital equipment needs, operating budget, revenue projections, cash flow needs, bookkeeping needs, and so forth.

The capital equipment needs of the project include basic office furniture and equipment. The initial costs will be approximately $10,000. More expensive pieces of equipment, such as copying machines, will be rented during the first year of operation.

The total operating budget, which follows, will be $151,620 for the first year of operation. Approximately 70 percent of that amount is fixed cost.

Salaries and fringe benefits	$94,800
Consultant (senior) 58 days @ $250 per day	14,500
Consultant (junior) 50 days @ $200 per day	10,000
Automobile (20,000 mile @ $0.25 per mile)	5,000
Consultant travel (10,000 miles @ $0.18 per mile)	1,800
Office space	6,000
Office equipment	1,500
Office furniture	1,500
Printing	2,000
Marketing	2,500
Legal	700
Accounting/bookkeeping	500

Insurance	500
Office supplies	2,000
Miscellaneous	2,000
Profit (8 percent of salaries $79,000)	6,330
	$151,620

The project will need to maintain an operating cash reserve of approximately $15,000. Bookkeeping will be handled internally.

The revenue projections are as follows:

Full-time members	$80,000
Part-time members	$40,000
Contracts	$20,000
Program income	$11,620
	$151,620

Assessment of Strengths and Weaknesses of Competitors

Organization	Strengths	Weaknesses
ORGANIZATION A: Probably the primary competitor at the present time; offers a broad variety of education and training services	Good leadership and professional staff	Limited staff with heavy work load
	Positive reputation; well known in hospitals throughout the region	A wide variety of services, and internal work in hospitals is presently a low priority
	Strong marketing capabilities	Heavy dependency on external consultants, limiting the profit on work delivered
	Success at offering conference-style management training programs	Extremely political organization, with much resistance and many turf issues involved with any new services
	A not-for-profit corporation	
ORGANIZATION B: A major competitor in the region; offers a wide variety of training programs for health care professionals (technical as well as management training)	Extensive package of hospital-related management training programs for hospital managers	Limited staff overburdened with heavy work load
		Currently at maximum capability
	Contracts with approximately 12 hospitals	Heavy dependency on external consultants, whose services present fee schedule can't handle

Organization	Strengths	Weaknesses
	Solid and broad base of funding	Limited to training services
	A very positive image in the hospital industry	
	Low fees	Political resistance to expansion
		Only a portion of the region as its defined market
ORGANIZATION C: A not-for-profit corporation that markets management and organizational development services for the local university	Talent pool of consultants with university base	Lack of hospital-based experience
	Active marketing	Lack of success in attempts to break into the hospital market
	A good image with industries in the region	High fee schedule
ORGANIZATION D: One of the better known private consulting firms used by hospitals to provide consultation regarding the management of union activities	Involvement with many hospitals in the region at the present time because of the high level of union activity	Bad reputation for management development activities
	A good reputation for union activity consultation	High fees
ORGANIZATION E: The statewide hospital association offers a broad range of services, including management and technical training programs	Politically strong relationship with hospitals	Very limited programming
	A full-time professional for management training programs	
ORGANIZATION F: A private consulting firm with owner as primary actor	Owner well known as a trainer in hospitals in the region	Broad market, including industry, government, education, and so forth
	Good training with solid materials	Works alone (limited resources)
		Pure training focus

NOTES

1. Tichy, N. A Social Network Perspective for Organizational Development. Unpublished paper prepared for the Graduate School of Business, Columbia University, New York.

2. Graig, D. *Hip Pocket Guide to Planning and Evaluation.* Austin, TX: Learning Concepts, 1978, pp. 139-40.

3. Morrisey, G. *Management by Objectives and Results.* Buena Vista, CA: MOR Associates, 1974, p. 39.

4. Maryland Hospital Education Institute. *1979 Annual Report.* Lutherville, MD: MHEI, 1979.

5. Two excellent references are McMillan, N. H. *Planning for Survival: A Handbook for Hospital Trustees.* Chicago: American Hospital Association, 1978, and Peters, J. P. *A Guide to Strategic Planning for Hospitals.* Chicago: American Hospital Association, 1979.

6. Bangs, David H. *Business Planning Guide.* Portsmouth, NH: Upstart Pub. Co., Inc., 1979.

Chapter 5

The Implementation Stage

The most difficult but often neglected work, formation, is completed. The implementation stage is a time to develop a sound governance and decision-making structure and to implement a plan to accomplish your mission, goals, and objectives.

Governance and Decision Making

One of the first steps in the implementation stage is the formation of a governance group and the development of decision-making policies and procedures. Two key questions must be answered:

- What form of governance group should you establish?
- Who will make what kinds of decisions using what process?

The number and types of decision-making groups will depend on the complexity of the organization and the types of services that it offers. Regardless of complexity, however, three groups appear to be essential: a centralized decision-making group, an advisory group, and a group responsible for coordinating communication with individual member organizations.

At a minimum, there must be a centralized decision-making body representing the member organizations. The task of this group is to define the mission of the organization; establish policy; make decisions regarding organizational structure, funding, staffing, and services; and address questions regarding project development, political issues, and other major problems. It is particularly important that the CEO of each member institution, or a senior manager with full decision-making authority, be involved in this group. The issues that need to addressed at this level require that the right people with power be sitting in the room.

In order to assure that programs and services are not developed in isolation and are responsive to the real needs of the member organizations, mechanisms for input from various layers of member organizations must be developed. The possibilities range from a multidisciplinary advisory group to address total shared service development to individual planning groups to develop specific programs and services for individual departments or professional disciplines. The effective use of these groups will improve the quality of services and increase the sense of "ownership" and support for the effort. It will also develop the informal relationship between hospital personnel and shared service staff.

Because the shared service will affect each member hospital, a clear internal decision-making process needs to be defined. The top management team should be directly involved in all major decision making. Managing of the day-to-day activities can be done in a variety of ways, depending on the particular hospital, its size, and the complexity of the work to be done. An internal education advisory group might be useful, or the entire process could be managed by the personnel administrator, HRD professional, or a key manager.

When providing services or programs within individual member hospitals, remember that the shared service invades the turf of the internal HRD department. The question should be raised constantly as to how the work can be done in such a manner as to enhance the position of the HRD department. The probability of success will be increased if the staff of the HRD department is comfortable that the activities will, in the long run, help it to accomplish its goals and objectives and develop its system. This is most likely to happen if the staff is fully involved in the decision-making process and can participate in the implementation of those decisions.

Although the number and types of formal decision-making groups are important to consider, it is also important to emphasize the role of the informal system and the need for informal meetings with key people in each organization. The support and loyalty that develop through informal relationships have a major impact on the degree to which people will act as advocates for project affairs, market programs internally, share their clinical expertise, and get people to attend programs.

Regardless of how many or what types of decision-making groups are set up, the right people must be included in the process. Appropriate membership might be identified by asking the following questions:

- Who has to be satisfied with the decisions?
- Who will have to implement the decisions?
- Who is going to have to manage the process?
- Who is going to be affected by the decisions?
- Who has valid and significant data?
- Who has sufficient power and influence to affect the decision either positively or negatively?

Once you can answer these questions, you can identify your members' needs. Involvement in the decision-making process can include making decisions, providing input prior to decisions, or being kept informed as to what decisions have been made and why. Appendix D provides a sample decision-making procedure adopted by the governance group of the Manchester Health Education Consortium in its early stages of development.

Another issue has to do with confidentiality. Because staff members of a shared service often have access to sensitive information about member institutions, it is recommended that clear procedures be developed to ensure that the integrity of any single institution or individual not be compromised. A sample of such a statement is shown in appendix E.

Development and Implementation of the Plan

The next step in the implementation stage is the development and implementation of the shared service plan. Two useful questions to consider during the completion of this step are:

- What guidelines should we follow?
- How do we overcome major barriers?

The potential for the types of programs or services that are offered in a shared HRD service is limited only by the defined mission and the organizational model that is chosen. These programs or services can include any or all of the organizational services outlined in figure 4, page 22. The implementation process for an individual program or service is simply a miniature repetition of the progress gone through for the implementation of the larger shared HRD service. You need to raise the same questions and apply the same principles. Successful implementation of programs is accomplished through effective application of the following guidelines:

- Careful diagnosis of the need for the program or service, the environment in which you expect to offer it, and the amount of support available
- Adequate information about the innovation, program, or services that you are going to implement, and anticipated questions and concerns that management and staff will have
- Development of sound strategies for developing support for your idea or proposal
- Development of a systematic approach to program implementation, monitoring, and evaluation.

If your diagnosis conducted during the pre-affiliation and formation stages of the process was done well, you established clear program directions for the implementation of the shared HRD service. However, you may still need to do more detailed assessment in specific program areas. The diagnostic process in many HRD efforts is frequently oversimplified because of the impatience of key decision makers who "want to see concrete results yesterday." These desired results can be accomplished only if programs and activities are based upon adequate diagnosis. You also should recognize that the diagnostic process itself helps build relationships between shared service staff and key people in member organizations.

Careful preparation and knowing your innovations (being well informed) will have a major impact on the successful implementation of programs or services within your shared HRD service. Use the following questions to determine how well you know what you are about to do. These questions are important because they help you focus on exactly what you want to do in response to specific HRD needs—for example, trustee education:

- What are your specific objectives (concrete measurable terms relating to quality, quantity, and time frame) for this particular service?
- What is the cost of implementing the program or service (including the costs of time, money, social status, and so forth)?
- What are the potential benefits, in both the short run and long run, for the organization and the individuals involved?
- How will the program or service make life easier or harder for people in member organizations?
- How much risk or uncertainty is involved?
- How complex is the program or service? If it is complex, can it be introduced in phases?
- How compatible is the program or service with the goals, values, priorities, and so forth of member organizations?

The effective manager of a shared service will constantly monitor the level of support of key individuals in the system for the projects, programs, or services. He will also have a conscious game plan or set of strategies for nurturing those who are actively supportive and for attempting to soften the impact of those who are actively offering resistance. The most common strategies to gain support from key people include:

- Inviting them to participate in decision making
- Emphasizing the impact (benefit) that the program will have on their priorities
- Requesting consultation from them and sharing information with them
- Showing connections between the program and the concepts, principles, and values to which those persons are committed
- Attempting to influence those who have contact with the key individuals
- Providing a clear analysis of the alternatives to the program, indicating the limitations of each compared with the program that you are recommending

Other principles include developing a sensitivity to key persons—their style and what approach they respond to, talking straight and being honest with them, not catching them by surprise, keeping them informed regarding problems that develop, choosing conflicts carefully, and respecting boundaries (such as continuing to test the important ones).

Because shared HRD services usually offer a variety of services and programs, you will need to develop an effective and efficient system to assure that all of the detailed activities are attended to in timely fashion. These details include a systematic approach to the design or development of individual programs and services, marketing, materials development, clear contracts and letters of agreement, arrangement of schedules and physical space, staffing, evaluation, record keeping, and consultation. Each manager has his or her own style, and, therefore, no one system can be universally applied to shared services. However, we strongly encourage you to develop an approach that will require you to develop a standardized written development plan for each program offered. This written plan will serve both as a guide and a checklist for all activities essential to successful programming. Your written plan should include the following: title, dates/time, location, instructor and qualifications, target audience, total instructional hours, description, objectives, outline schedule, teaching methods, material and equipment, space requirements, work to be done before program, continuing education requirements, evaluation requirements, financial analysis (projected costs and income), contracts/letters of agreement, and checklists for the coordinator.

During stages 1 and 2, you were careful to analyze those factors that could affect the successful implementation of a shared HRD service. In step 12, those that have not surfaced are certain to appear; at the national research conference mentioned in the first chapter, participants identified the problems most troublesome to them during the implementation stage, and listed successful strategies they had used to combat each. A summary of this discussion is presented in table 2, pages 29-31.

You have now melded needs with programming objectives and, barring unforeseen circumstances, have agreed to proceed with full implementation and integration of resources. You also know how you want to do what you need to do. The most critical leadership task during the implementation stage is to attain concrete results that develop credibility in the shared service and inspire confidence that it will succeed. You need to establish an appropriate course of action for yourself and others to achieve established goals, make proper assignment of personnel and appropriate use of resources, establish procedures or systems to monitor or control program development implementation, and evaluate results and make necessary adjustments. At this point, you need a good sense of detail, a high level of perseverance, and the ability to manage within a fairly ambiguous and stressful environment.

Chapter 6

The Stabilization and Renewal Stage

The final stage in the development of a shared HRD service requires an honest appraisal of the benefits, successes, failures, strengths, and weaknesses of the effort. Appraisal requires answers to four basic questions:

1. What are we trying to do (goals and objectives)?
2. Did it get done (identification and collection of data)?
3. What do the data show (analysis)?
4. What are our next steps?

Two steps in this process occur simultaneously, interacting in a cyclical fashion: Individual members must carefully assess the benefits that they are receiving from the shared services, and they must clarify their expectations for future services in a formal appraisal. During the pre-affiliation stage, questions were raised about the fit between the needs of an individual institution and the services provided by the shared service. The question now is whether or not the fit resulted as expected. At the same time, one must appraise the total shared service organization itself to determine its level of effectiveness in accomplishing its mission, goals, and objectives. Only when success occurs on both levels can one claim true success. Then you can decide on your future directions, whether that be maintenance of the status quo, expansion, reduction in service, or the creation of a very different organization.

Assessing Benefits to the Institution

In the continual appraisal of a shared service's value to your institution, you will be concerned about several key issues: Did you get what you wanted? What were the payoffs and costs? Which problems were most troublesome? What changes would you like to see?

Frequently, the weakest link in the development of shared HRD services is the individual institution's lack of clarity about its specific needs and expectations. The individual institution should be particularly concerned about the real results arising from participation in the project, the quality of programs and services, the quantity of services received, a cost-benefit analysis, the ability to influence decisions related to services offered and future directions, and the quality of relationships between individuals and groups.

In brief, you should find an improvement in the state of affairs between "what is" and "what ought to be" that you examined in the pre-affiliation stage. These questions need to be raised at various levels of the organization. In chapters 2 and 4, you were asked to identify the key actors or constituency groups. You need to collect data from all of them, making careful note of any differing perceptions. Support is needed

55

at all layers of the organization, and it is not adequate to satisfy one group and ignore the others. It also helps to refer back to the rational, political, and normative motivations for participation and assess the degree to which each of those needs were met. Too frequently, evaluation is limited to the rational level and ignores the payoffs and problems that may have been experienced in the normative and political domains.

Internal Mechanisms for Ongoing Appraisal

Appraisal is frequently the weakest part of most shared HRD services. Yet, an effective appraisal effort provides the opportunity to improve the quality of the services being offered and provides objective data for developing new services. The extent of an appraisal will vary tremendously, depending on its particular purpose. When designing an appraisal, you might consider the following questions:

- What do you want the evaluation to show, and how soon?
- What data are necessary?
- What are the most effective and efficient methods to collect data?
- What do you need to know, in what areas, and what is the priority of each of those areas?
- What do you want to do with the resultant information?

Appraisal as a process is most helpful when it is an active consideration in each of the four stages and 17 steps. Used in this way, appraisal becomes a tool that can help to upgrade quality and improve programs while they are in progress, rather than an uninvolved and usually harsh judgment pronounced when the work is finished and when few, if any, changes can be made.

There is no right way to appraise; how you get information and analyze it will depend on your needs and those of the people with whom you are working. People perform appraisals every day. The task in an organizational setting is to do that evaluation in a more systematic way so that the results might be used more consciously and effectively. If managed well, the stabilization and renewal stage:

- Demonstrates a shared commitment to delivering predicted results, thus strengthening credibility
- Provides a process for critical examination of the services offered by the project and provides a data base for establishing new directions
- Provides an opportunity to assess the strengths and weaknesses of the organization
- Enables member institutions to decide whether to expand, maintain, or reduce individual or collective participation in the project

Decisions about the Future

Inevitably, during the stabilization and renewal stage you must make a decision about whether to seek fuller integration of resources, maintain the status quo, alter the plan, or terminate the agreement. Essentially, you must answer four questions:

- Do you wish to receive the same kind and amount of services?
- Should new activities be initiated?
- Do you wish to continue in the project?
- What kinds of changes need to be made in the ways you are interacting with the shared service organization?

Clarifying Expectations

The baseline for formal evaluation of a shared service is the mission and goals established during step 8. You need to conduct a careful analysis of each objective, the degree to which it was accomplished, and any difficulties encountered along the way. It is essential that this process be conducted in an honest and forthright manner, with input from key parties. The purpose is not to assign blame, but to get an objective picture of what actually happened in order to make decisions about the future. Table 3, pages 58-62, displays a sample evaluation of objectives for a four-hospital shared HRD service that covers 12 different areas from administration through evaluation. It serves as one model you could consider. However, the overall evaluation should rarely be based simply on whether or not the established objectives are accomplished. Other factors to be considered include:

- The reasons for success or failure
- The proper allocation of time and resource
- The type and difficulty of objectives
- The creativity in overcoming obstacles
- Additional objectives undertaken
- The manner in which problems/crises were handled
- Good management practices

Allocation of Resources

Although in this step you focus on the total effort, you need to look at how resources were allocated among institutions, because the equity issue is always on the surface. This is particularly important if organizational models are based on funding mechanisms that include membership fees. Each member expects to receive its equitable share of the services provided compared with its investment of dollars.

Figure 11, page 63, demonstrates one approach to this dilemma, a comparison of contact hours received by member institutions during three years of operation. People tend to be motivated by comparing how they are doing in relation to others. More than one CEO has responded to such a chart with statements such as "I can assure you that we will bring up our figures next year!" It is also helpful to show comparative data from one year to the next. This enables you to pick up changing patterns with an individual institution.

Analysis of Costs

One of the primary rational motives for a shared HRD service is the potential dollar savings that are realized. It is particularly useful to do a cost-benefit analysis for each service offered to determine whether there was an adequate savings or return on investment. It is fairly simple to determine the unit cost of individual services and compare that figure to what it would cost to purchase comparable services from other providers. It is more difficult to determine how much, if any, money was saved by the institution as a result of the services received.

Evaluation of Specific Project Elements

An example of the evaluation of a specific project element is displayed in table 4, page 64. This appraisal plan outlines the levels of assessment that could occur if a shared HRD service wanted to fully evaluate each institution's performance management systems (performance appraisal, goal setting, reward practices).

Planning for the Future

You are now in a position to revise or develop a plan of action for the future. Before putting this plan together, however, you might ask yourself the following questions:

- What are the major threats and opportunities for the future?
- What impact have key individuals and constituency groups had on the project?
- What are the major forces that have had an impact on the organization during the past year? What forces are likely to be present in the coming year?
- Have there been any inconsistencies between our activities and our defined mission?
- How are we doing in relation to our competition?

Table 3. Evaluation of Objectives

Objective	Status	Result
1. To comply with all fiscal and federal guidelines	Accomplished	
2. To present a formal recommendation to the executive committee by 12/31/80, regarding an appropriate organizational structure that will enable the consortium to continue its operation in the fourth year	Accomplished	The member hospitals have created a not-for-profit corporation that will carry on all consortium activities once the IRS tax-exempt status is approved. Projected time frame: 9/81
Consortium Development		
1. To retain Hospitals A, B, C, D as full members	Accomplished	All members have continued for three years; one hospital, however, will not be continuing as a full member in the fourth year due to corporate restrictions.
2. To expand project activities to include at least three partial members by 9/30/80	Partially accomplished	Political concerns have slowed down all expansion efforts; proposals regarding an option for contracted services were mailed to three medical hospitals in the region. One has entered into an agreement, one is still undecided, and the third has responded negatively.
3. To implement an expansion plan, according to schedule, and resource allocations as recommended by the executive committee	To be accomplished	By the end of June, proposals will be mailed to all health care agencies in the region regarding options for contracted services.
Finances		
1. To manage funds in accordance with preestablished guidelines at a cost not to exceed eight staff days	Accomplished	
2. To expand budget funds within plus or minus 5% of the budget for line items and to request no more than two budget changes	Accomplished	Only one formal budget revision has been submitted.
3. To establish a system for the financial management of the consortium in the fourth year by 5/1/80	To be accomplished	The fiscal aspects of the project will be managed by project staff with the assistance of staff from member hospitals.
4. To raise a minimum of $24,391 in hospital assessments during 1980-81	Accomplished	
5. To earn at least $10,000 in program and other income by 6/30/81	Surpassed objective	The project will have grossed more than $13,000 in the program and other income by 6/30/81.

Table 3. Evaluation of Objectives (continued)

Objective	Status	Result
Needs Assessment		
1. To complete a full needs assessment of any new member institution within two months of admission at a cost not to exceed seven staff days and $150 per hospital	Not applicable	No new members were accepted during the third year.
2. To assess the training and development needs of member hospitals on an ongoing basis	Accomplished	Three member hospitals conducted simple needs assessments regarding management training needs with consortium assistance. Consortium staff also conducted in-depth assessments to provide baseline data for developing management training programs at Hospitals C and D.
3. To meet with the interhospital planning groups listed below once every three months to identify the education needs of individual departments. The groups are to include: Coordinators of nursing in-service education, Chief lab technicians, Chief x-ray technicians, Chairmen of safety committees, Dietitians, Executive secretaries, Infection control nurses, Medical emergency planning committee, Medical records administrators, Psychiatric emergency committee	Accomplished	The Safety Committee, Infection Control Committee, medical records administrators, and secretaries met only once, which appeared to be sufficient. Additional committees focusing on patient education, pharmacology, and legal issues were established.
Education Programs		
1. To provide 25,000 trainee hours for educational programs by 6/30/81, at a cost not to exceed $10,000 and 206 professional man-days; programs will meet these guidelines:		
a. Programming will reach 1,500 participants		Programs reached 2,896 participants
b. Programming will reach 75% of employee groups		Programs reached 77% of employee groups.
c. Unit costs will not exceed an average of $2.50 per trainee hour.		Unit costs averaged $2.49.
d. Participant reaction to programs will average 5.0 on a 7.0 scale (3.0 on a 4.0 scale).		Participant reaction averaged 5.1 on a scale of 6.
e. 75% of participants queried in follow-up activities will agree, measured as 3.0 on a 4.0 scale (5.0 on a 7.0 scale), that they were able to apply their learnings on the job and that there was an observable increase in job performance.		Follow-up evaluations have not been conducted except for management training programs. Regarding ability to apply learning on the job, satisfaction with the average management training is 4.6 on a scale of 6.

(continued on next page)

Table 3. Evaluation of Objectives (continued)

Objective	Status	Result
f. 50% of supervisors queried will indicate, measured as 2.5 on a 4.0 scale (5.0 on a 7.0 scale), that the job performance of their employees improved after participation in programs.		Follow-up evaluations have not been conducted with supervisors.
2. To conduct at least two priority programs within each participating hospital by 6/30/80 at a cost not to exceed the educational program budget and allotted staff days	Accomplished with three of the four members	All but Hospital D have received a minimum of two priority programs.
3. To continue development and offering of core programs by:	Partially accomplished	The three modules have been developed, but the program was delayed awaiting approval of the first two modules for certification by intensive care unit nursing personnel. The first module was completed in 5/81. It will be repeated in the fall followed by the other two modules.
a. Completing the development of the three modular coronary care series by 9/1/80, and completing the first module by 12/1/80, at a cost not to exceed $500 and three professional man-days; the second module by 3/1/81, at a cost not to exceed $500 and three professional man-days; the third module by 6/1/81, at a cost not to exceed $500 and two professional man-days		
b. Completing the development of the respiratory care program for nursing personnel by 9/1/80, and conducting the program three times by 6/30/81, at a cost not to exceed $800 and five professional man-days	Partially accomplished	A basic program (18 hours) was conducted twice; the advanced program (18 hours) was developed but not offered due to personal issues relating to the instructor. It will be offered in the fall.

Management Education

Objective	Status	Result
1. To continue to develop and implement the management training system program including:	Accomplished	Member hospitals received the following number of internal programs: Hospital A,6; Hospital B,3; Hospital C,1; and Hospital D,1.
a. At least two management training programs in Hospitals A, B, and D, and one in Hospital C by 6/30/80, at a cost not to exceed $800 and 52 professional man-days		
b. Two central offerings of Introduction to Hospital Supervision, Training and Developing Employees, and Orienting Employees, by 6/30/80, at a cost not to exceed $600 and 40 professional man-days	Partially accomplished	Introduction to Hospital Supervision and Training and Developing Employees were offered once. Orienting Employees was never offered due to other priorities.

Table 3. Evaluation of Objectives (continued)

Objective	Status	Result
c. At least six special-interest seminars for managers in member hospitals during 1979-80 at a cost not to exceed $200 and three professional man-days	Revised	Rather than a series of two-hour programs, several special-interest, daylong programs were offered on topics including legal aspects of management, rate setting, and managing stress (cancelled due to lack of support).
2. To cosponsor a pilot training program with the American Hospital Association for trainers to implement the guidelines for establishing a cost containment committee by 12/1/80, at a cost not to exceed $300 and eight professional man-days	Tabled	The executive committee tabled this objective due to the projected costs involved.
3. To develop a 12-hour pilot team-building workshop to assist in the development of existing management teams in member institutions by 9/1/81, at a cost not to exceed $200 and 10 professional man-days	Accomplished	This program was offered at Hospital A in the fall.
Trainer Development		
1. To conduct a minimum of four full days of trainer development activities by 6/30/81, at a cost not to exceed $500 and 18 professional man-days.	Not Accomplished	The first two days of this program were scheduled for January and delayed until May because of attempts to cosponsor the program with other key agencies. The program was ultimately cancelled.
Consultation		
1. To respond to all reasonable requests for consultation in training and development activities from personnel of member institutions at a cost not to exceed 36 staff days	Accomplished	Member hospitals received the targeted quantity of consultation.
2. To meet at least once each month with the education committees of member institutions at a cost not to exceed 12 staff days	Tabled	The education and training committees of member hospitals were generally considered to be ineffective mechanisms for decision making. Major decisions were made with the senior administration of member hospitals.
Resource Clearinghouse		
1. To respond to all requests for training and development resources within five staff days	Accomplished	
2. To develop and expand the learning resource files to 75 content areas by 6/1/80	Accomplished	
3. To maintain files on all programs conducted or sponsored in 1979-80	Accomplished	
Staff Development		
1. To develop MOR agreements with each staff person by 7/15/80, at a cost not to exceed five staff days	Accomplished	Clear standards were established for all objectives determined and responsibilities assigned.

(continued on next page)

Table 3. Evaluation of Objectives (continued)

Objective	Status	Result
2. To provide each staff member a minimum of 10 days of professional development training (five for administrative secretary) at a cost not to exceed $1,500 and 25 staff days	Partially Accomplished	
3. To hold at least two staff meetings per month to review project activities and progress against objectives at a cost not to exceed nine staff days	Accomplished	
System Coordination		
1. To coordinate consortium activities with the efforts of other institutions and agencies in the region so that there are not justifiable complaints of duplication as judged by the executive committee	Ongoing effort	
2. To distribute at least 400 copies of *Interchange* by the fourth of each month at a cost not to exceed $400 and 12 professional man-days	Accomplished	500 copies of *Interchange* are distributed on a monthly basis.
3. To update the union list of learning resources and audiovisuals available in the consortium office and hospitals on a monthly basis at a cost not to exceed $100 and three professional man-days	Ongoing effort	
4. To update the union list of journals and periodicals available in the consortium office and hospitals by 11/1/81, at a cost not to exceed $300 and three professional man-days	Tabled	Due to the availability of other union lists, this objective was tabled.
5. To assist the interhospital task force to assess the potential for sharing of library and audiovisual learning resources and prepare a report for the executive committee by 9/1/80	Tabled	Due to other priorities this objective was tabled.
Evaluation		
1. To prepare a full evaluation report for the third year by 6/30/81 at a cost not to exceed four staff days	Accomplished	
2. To prepare a report on consortium activity in each member hospital by 4/1/80, at a cost not to exceed eight staff days	Accomplished	
3. To prepare a full evaluation on the activities of the consortium during its first three years of operation by 6/30/81	Accomplished	

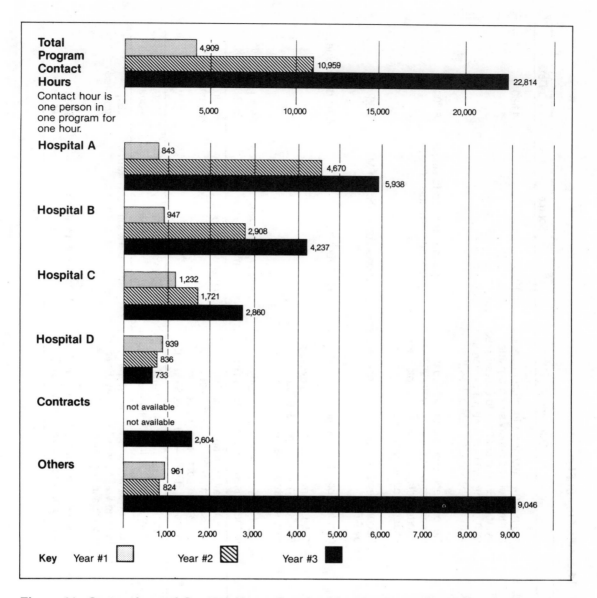

Figure 11. Comparison of Contact Hours Received by Member Institutions in 3 Years

Table 4. Evaluation of Specific Project Elements

Area of Performance	Outcome	Source	Date
Program implementation	1. Train 100+ managers in initial cycle of midlevel and supervisory programs by 10/31/80 at a cost not to exceed $660 ($70 direct; $590 indirect) per person and with an absenteeism rate of less than 5%.	HRD records	11/80
	2. Recommend changes in individual hospital reward systems by 5/23/80; conduct diagnoses by 4/81; implement changes as scheduled.	Reports submitted to senior management team (SMT)	6/80
	3. Recommend changes in personnel systems by 6/6/80.	Reports submitted to SMT	7/80
	4. Conduct physician program.	HRD records	(to be determined)
	5. Total estimated cost is not to exceed $84,500 ($18,000 direct, $66,500 indirect) through 9/80.		
	6. Meet all other deadlines as outlined in the revised implementation plan.	HRD cost sheets, implementation plan	10/81 3/82
Cost comparison	7. Conduct all training at total cost of less than 50% of fair market value (pegged at cost of $1,350 per person in market; direct—$70 in vs. $900 out).	HRD cost sheets	11/80, repeated
Participant reaction (immediate)	8. Attain a level of 1.0+ on E-7 and other evaluation instruments.	E-7 evaluations	11/80, repeated
Participant evaluation (3 to 6 months after training)	9. 90% of participants will report that training was "useful" and that they have "used the skills."	Participant follow-up form	5/81, repeated
	10. 60% will report three tangible outcomes as a result of using the skills.	Participant follow-up form	5/81, repeated

Table 4. Evaluation of Specific Project Elements (continued)

Area of Performance	Outcome	Source	Date
Supervisor's evaluation (3 to 6 months after training)	11. 80% of supervisors will report that training was "useful" and that it was "used" by their subordinates; 60% will report that subordinates conducted more "performance-related discussions."	Supervisor's follow-up form	5/81, repeated
	12. 50% of supervisors will report three "tangible" results achieved by supervisor's use of the skills.	Supervisor's follow-up form	5/81, repeated
Cost-benefit analysis (subjective; 12 months after training)	13. 60% of participants will report a return on investment (ROI*) of 3:1+ (based on subjective data); 50% of superiors will confirm participant reports.	ROI appraisal form	10/81, repeated
SMT appraisal (subjective; after second year of project)	14. SMT will confirm that consortium helped each institution achieve an ROI of 3:1 after two years of project.	SMT assessment meeting	3/1/82
Cost-benefit analysis (against targeted objectives in pilot departments)	15. 60% of departments demonstrate an average ROI of 3:1 or greater	Interviews with pilot departments	11/81

*ROI based on documentation of "measurable" results by comparing costs versus benefits. The measurable costs and benefits will be based on hard and soft data agreed to by boss, subordinate, and top management group or subgroup.

Assessing Programming

Two key issues that commonly arise at this stage are the questions of appropriate size and scope of programming. Participants at the 1977 National Research Conference on Shared Education Services identified lists of indicators to decide about these factors.

Indicators that a service may be too large include the realization that the service costs more to maintain than you can make in revenues, an inability to keep commitments or provide supporting services for programs, duplication, lack of an accurate assessment of the impact of efforts, decreased utilization of services, the feeling that too many supervisors exist and that too much time is spent keeping everyone informed, large committees, frequent breakdowns in communication, a loose sense of mission and loose coordination of staff, failing programs, complaints that needs are not being met, lack of service utilization by members, and complaints by staff that they are overloaded.

Indicators that a service may be too small include findings that you are spending most of your time on administration rather than on education, data suggesting that the service costs more to maintain than you make in revenues, the feeling that you are swamped with work, numerous questions about what you're doing, inability to meet needs and reasonable requests, difficulty identifying resources, a lack of basic strategies concerning needs assessment and evaluation, inadequate resources including faculty, funding, and audiovisuals, lack of services to share, and a realization that potential resources and/or members are not being tapped.

Likewise, indicators signaling problems in the scope of programming were developed. Potential signs of program overload include complaints of administrators and managers that there are too many programs, numerous long-distance crisis calls to order materials, poor enrollment, scheduling complaints of overload, internal frustration, program cancellations, poor program evaluations, use of the same target audience over and over, poorly planned curriculum, an exhausted staff, not keeping to timetables and complaining of insufficient time to research the need for programs under development, lack of time to apply for accreditation, mechanical breakdowns, and late mailings.

Evidence of insufficient programming includes many identified current needs, long waiting lists for future programs, findings that inappropriate groups are taking courses, problems with accreditation surveys, lack of interest, flagging support, complaints that programs are too general, too broad, or not specific enough, and poorly defined needs.

Recycling

The "final" step in the stabilization and renewal stage is a recycling of the process, usually beginning with the development and implementation of a shared service plan (step 12). Generally, you will need to redefine the level or type of service you deliver or produce a new plan. On occasion, however, you may discover that you want to rewrite your mission statement (step 11), redesign the organization (step 9), or even repeat such pre-affiliation steps as appraising internal HRD needs and readiness, determining environmental readiness, and initiating discussions with key leaders (steps 1, 2, and 4).

Such activities need not consume the time they may have at first. You now have the experience and knowledge to make an informed decision based upon valid data.

The primary leadership skills needed during the stabilization and renewal stage include the ability to evaluate program activities, analyze problems, generate imaginative and innovative approaches, and take calculated risks in order to achieve maximum benefits from decisions and activities. Stabilization also requires leaders who build systems that result in efficiency, coach and challenge staff to develop new skills, and develop broad bases of support through linkages with key individuals and organizations.

Appendix A

Management Skills Inventory

What Is the Management Skills Inventory?

The purpose of this inventory is to help hospitals identify the most critical development needs of themselves and their subordinate managers/supervisors. The task is to identify three specific skills each manager will improve or develop during the year. The process is outlined below.

After each manager completes the inventory for subordinates and develops one for himself or herself, Human Resource Development (HRD) will compile an institutional profile for presentation to the senior management group. That group will use the profile to plan the hospital's management development programs for the year. HRD will assume responsibility for developing and conducting selected programs, for helping managers find ways to develop skills in areas HRD cannot cover, and for coordinating efforts to evaluate the impact of the program.

How to Complete the Skills Inventory

1. Meet with your subordinate managers/supervisors to explain the purpose of the inventory and agree to a process for completing it.
2. Complete the skills inventory for your subordinate and have him/her prepare a self-inventory using the same instrument:
   a. Review each of the skills listed in column A of the inventory and then, in section 7, list additional skills peculiar to your/your subordinate's job.
   b. If you are appraising yourself, use column B to assess your present level of competence in handling each particular skill. Use the scale that follows below. If the skill is not applicable, write N/A in the blank. Your supervisor will provide ratings for column C.
   c. If you are appraising a subordinate manager or supervisor, use column C, following the instructions above. Your subordinate will provide ratings for column B. Use the following ratings:

5 Outstanding	An exceptional performer. Could teach others this skill.
4 Highly skilled	A real strength. No further development needed.
3 Generally competent	Competence level is adequate for the job, but fine-tuning would improve performance.
2 Limited competence	Often an area of difficulty; or, an area of little experience. Development needed.

| 1 Minimal competence | A definite problem area; or, an area of very limited experience and training. Development essential. |

3. Meet to integrate your analyses. Record both sets of responses on your form and compare analyses.

4. Circle potential developmental needs. Needs may be single skills, such as handling disciplinary problems; clusters of skills, such as resolving conflict downward, upward, and laterally; or entire skill areas, such as performance management. You may circle those skills rated 1 or 2 by either party, those rated differently by each of you, or those rated 3 which, if improved, would make a real difference. You may also circle items that are handled well enough for the present job but need to be developed further before promotion or increased responsibility.

5. Agree on two or three developmental goals. After reviewing those skills you've circled, use column D, and the scale below, to jointly assess how critical each skill is to the particular job you're assessing. Then, select your goals, rating them as follows:

3 Critical	Essential to develop or improve this skill now because it is so critical to performance.
2 High priority	Not as critical as some skills, but should be kept high on the list.
1 Low priority	Can wait, but needs to be developed; or, not really important for this job.

6. Write a development plan (see sample format on page 72) that includes development needs, the commitments of the supervisor, and plans for reviewing progress. These questions may help you develop that plan:
   - What training programs or other educational experiences would be useful?
   - What activities is my supervisor involved in that I could be doing to help me learn this skill?
   - What activities am I doing that I could delegate to help my subordinate develop this skill?
   - What books, articles, or other self-learning materials would help in developing this skill?
   - What barriers might prevent me from improving this skill? How can I overcome them?

7. Communicate those plans to HRD. HRD will develop an institutional profile. Your responses will remain confidential, but will appear in summary form along with those of other managers and supervisors at the hospital.

A	B	C	D
		Supervisor's	Relative
Skills and Activity Area	**Self-Rating**	**Rating**	**Importance**

Section 1: One-on-One Supervision
1. Dealing with employee performance and/or work habit problems
2. Dealing with grievances and complaints of employees and/or patients
3. Handling disciplinary problems

A	B	C	D
		Supervisor's	**Relative**
Skills and Activity Area	**Self-Rating**	**Rating**	**Importance**

4. Delegating responsibility to subordinates appropriate to their abilities
5. Handling emotional situations and strong feelings
6. Maintaining and enhancing the self-esteem of subordinates
7. Providing subordinates with information they need to do their jobs
8. Introducing and overcoming resistance to change
9. Gaining acceptance as a manager or supervisor from employees
10. Involving subordinates appropriately in decision making and planning

Section 2: Task Effectiveness
1. Laying out day-to-day work so that employees can get things done efficiently
2. Analyzing work procedures and systems and making necessary improvements
3. Developing, monitoring, and controlling operating budgets
4. Managing the time of self and subordinates efficiently
5. Developing plans for projects and long-term assignments
6. Setting priorities and meeting deadlines

Section 3: Performance Management
1. Setting performance goals and/or job expectations
2. Communicating goals/expectations to subordinates
3. Designing job descriptions as the job changes
4. Providing timely and specific day-to-day feedback to employees
5. Conducting effective performance appraisal interviews for development/periodic review purposes

A	B	C	D
		Supervisor's	Relative
Skills and Activity Area	Self-Rating	Rating	Importance

6. Conducting merit review interviews

7. Administering the merit pool equitably and efficiently

Section 4: Selection, Orientation, and Training

1. Conducting selection interviews to make sound hiring decisions.

2. Orienting the employee to the job and using the probationary period well

3. Training the employee to do the job he/she was hired to do

4. Coaching and developing employees in nonsupervisory positions

5. Coaching and developing subordinate supervisors

Section 5: Conflict Resolution and Managing Inter-departmental/Unit Relations

1. Resolving dysfunctional conflict upward—with superior(s) and/or the organization

2. Resolving dysfunctional conflict sideways—with peers and other departments/units in the hospital

3. Resolving conflict downward— with subordinates

4. Functioning as a third party or mediator to help others resolve conflicts

5. Getting cooperation and action from people not under his/her control

Section 6: Communication and Interpersonal Effectiveness

1. Demonstrating an appropriate level of assertiveness in given situations.

2. Listening and responding to superiors and peers

3. Listening and responding with empathy to subordinates

4. Planning, conducting, and following up meetings

A	B	C	D
		Supervisor's	Relative
Skills and Activity Area	Self-Rating	Rating	Importance

5. Developing effective teamwork within/between work groups under his/her control
6. Writing effective letters, memos, and reports
7. Making effective verbal presentations to superiors, subordinates, and/or users

Section 7: Technical Skills/ Administering Hospital Policies and Procedures

1. Keeping up to date on technical knowledge in his/her field, and communicating implications to superior(s) and subordinates
2. Administering personnel policies
3. Preventing accidents and unsafe work practices on the job
4. Managing the union contract appropriately
5. Other skills needed by this manager/supervisor not listed here (list and rate as above):
   a.
   b.
   c.
   d.

Section 8: Leadership Effectiveness and Flexibility

1. Understanding the appropriateness of using alternative leadership styles in different situations
2. Demonstrating an ability to adapt leadership behaviors to the situation at hand
3. Managing effectively in situations where multicultural differences (race, sex, age, ethnic background, class, and so on) may affect task accomplishment negatively
4. Gaining acceptance from peers and higher levels in the hospitals
5. Demonstrating an adeptness at organizational politics
6. Understanding and using his/her power and authority constructively
7. Seeking feedback and self- and organizational improvements

A	B	C	D
Skills and Activity Area	**Self-Rating**	**Supervisor's Rating**	**Relative Importance**

8. Identifying problems, separating causes from symptoms, evaluating evidence, weighing alternatives, and implementing alternative solutions
9. Handling emergencies, crises, and the unexpected without drastically upsetting normal operations or employee stability
10. Thinking of creative ideas and innovative solutions when needed
11. Managing his/her own stress level and that of subordinates to prevent negative personal or organizational consequences

Development Plan

MANAGER:

DATE:

UNIT:

DEVELOPMENT NEEDS:

    1. Need:

       Steps:

    2. Need:

       Steps:

    3. Need:

       Steps:

COMMITMENTS OF SUPERVISOR:

PLANS FOR REVIEWING PROGRESS:

Appendix B

Survey Tool of MHEC

Name of Hospital:
    Hospital A   _____
    Hospital B   _____
    Hospital C   _____
    Hospital D   _____
    Hospital E   _____

Job Classification:
    Department head/service chief   _____
    Supervisor   _____
    Nonsupervisory employee   _____

Sex:
    Male   _____
    Female   _____

Tenure:
    0-6 years on job in this hospital   _____
    More than 6 years on job in this hospital   _____

Age:
    Under 25   _____
    25-34   _____
    35-44   _____
    45-54   _____
    55-64   _____
    65 or over   _____

Education:
    Less than high school diploma   _____
    High school diploma   _____
    2-3 years associate degree or diploma   _____
    Some college   _____
    College degree   _____
    Graduate work or degree   _____

Job Status:
    Full-time   _____
    Part-time   _____

Service Area:
    _____   Administrative services
                     (executive, fiscal, EDP, personnel, public relations, purchasing, and so on)

_____ Nursing services
_____ Plant operations/maintenance services
(engineering, maintenance, housekeeping, laundry, and so on)
_____ Professional care services (nonnursing)
(all other services, for example, dietetics, records, radiology, and
so on)

Name of Department: _____

1. Have you ever been a participant in in-service education programs (other than regular academic courses and orientation programs) during the past 24 months? Yes_____ No_____

Instructions:
If you responded yes to question 1, please answer questions 2-4; if you responded no, move directly to question 5 and continue from there.

2. How many training programs have you taken in each of the following categories during the past 24 months? (Insert the number of programs—up to 9—in the blank; do not count one course into more than one category.)
   a. Training to improve your performance in a specific job _____
   b. Training to keep in step with changes in your field, changes in organization, or changes in technology _____
   c. Training for future development for advancement in your organization _____

3. How many hours of actual instruction time did you spend in these programs? (Circle total for all programs attended.)
   1-2 hours   3-4   5-6   7-8   9-10   11-12   13 plus

4. Below is a list of statements about the quality and usefulness of the training you have received. Circle the number on the scale that corresponds to your opinion. If, for some reason, you cannot make a judgment, circle the 0, which means "not applicable."

	Disagree	Neutral	Agree	N/A
a. I am satisfied with the training I have received.	1 2 3	4 5	6 7	0
b. I would recommend that others in my position take advantage of similar opportunities.	1 2 3	4 5	6 7	0
c. I am satisfied with the amount of participation I have had in selecting the courses I attended.	1 2 3	4 5	6 7	0
d. The purpose of the training I received is clear to me.	1 2 3	4 5	6 7	0
e. The programs I attended were adequate to fulfill my specific needs.	1 2 3	4 5	6 7	0

5. Have you been given any additional responsibilities in the past 24 months? Yes_____ No_____
   If yes, did you receive adequate preparation and training? Yes_____ No_____

6. Below is a list of factors that would encourage or discourage you from voluntarily participating in educational programs. For each item, please circle the number that expresses your opinion.

	Would Encourage	Would Discourage	Would Have No Effect
a. Programs held outside regular working hours	1	2	3
b. Program held in evening	1	2	3
c. Program located in my hospital	1	2	3

d. Program located in another regional hospital	1	2	3
e. College credit or C.E.U.s offered	1	2	3
f. Released from work, with pay, to attend	1	2	3
g. Promotion opportunities tied to successful completion	1	2	3
h. Increased responsibility tied to participation	1	2	3
i. Written test or other examination required	1	2	3
j. Program located at or conducted by outside educational institution	1	2	3
k. Overnight stay involved	1	2	3
l. Travel time each way exceeds 60 minutes	1	2	3

7. Below is a list of statements about training, education, and opportunity for growth and development in this hospital. Read each statement and decide how you feel about it. Circle the number on the scale that corresponds to your opinion. If the statements do not apply to you, or if you have insufficient information available to make a judgment, circle the 0, which means "not applicable."

	Disagree		Neutral		Agree			N/A
a. I have been able to attend the programs I wanted to attend	1	2	3	4	5	6	7	0
b. My supervisor is committed to my training and development	1	2	3	4	5	6	7	0
c. Hospital policy promotes my training and development	1	2	3	4	5	6	7	0
d. I am receiving the training necessary to do my present job properly	1	2	3	4	5	6	7	0
e. I am receiving the training needed for future advancement	1	2	3	4	5	6	7	0
f. The counseling I receive from my supervisor concerning my own training and development is adequate	1	2	3	4	5	6	7	0
g. I receive adequate, timely information about what training opportunities are available	1	2	3	4	5	6	7	0
h. The selection of employees for attendance in courses is fair and without bias	1	2	3	4	5	6	7	0
i. The people who get promotions around here usually deserve them	1	2	3	4	5	6	7	0
j. There are many opportunities around here for people who want to get ahead	1	2	3	4	5	6	7	0

8. Below is a list of areas in which the consortium and your education staff can offer education and training programs to help you learn about certain aspects of your work. Please read the list carefully. For each item indicate on a scale of one (1) to five (5) how important it is for you to learn more in that particular category. Circle the number that comes closest to expressing your opinion.

	Very Important			Unimportant	
a. Improving technical job skills	1	2	3	4	5
b. Knowing more about the operation of the hospital and the department	1	2	3	4	5

c. Understanding the work of other departments	1	2	3	4	5
d. Utilizing new equipment	1	2	3	4	5
e. Understanding new regulations and procedures affecting jobs	1	2	3	4	5
f. Applying the fundamentals of aseptic technique	1	2	3	4	5
g. Developing better relations with fellow employees	1	2	3	4	5
h. Developing better relations with supervisors	1	2	3	4	5
i. Developing better relations with patients and their families	1	2	3	4	5
j. Developing better relations with other departments	1	2	3	4	5
k. Handling emergencies	1	2	3	4	5
l. Improving basic skills such as reading and writing communications	1	2	3	4	5
m. Coping with the emotional aspects of working in a hospital	1	2	3	4	5
n. Preparing self for promotion	1	2	3	4	5
o. Correcting weaknesses pointed out in performance appraisals	1	2	3	4	5

Are there any items you would like to add to this list?

_____

_____

_____

	Very Well	Moderately Well	Fairly Well	Not Well At All
9. When you first came to work here: (circle the appropriate number)				
a. How well were you instructed regarding your immediate job duties and responsibilities?	1	2	3	4
b. How well were you told about working conditions, salary, and employee benefits?	1	2	3	4
c. How well were you taught about the functions of departments other than your own?	1	2	3	4
d. How well were you trained to perform any new tasks you were assigned?	1	2	3	4

10. Below is a list of statements about relations between supervisors and employees. Circle the number on the scale for each item that corresponds to your opinion.

	Disagree			Neutral			Agree
a. My supervisor gives us credit and praise for work well done	1	2	3	4	5	6	7
b. My supervisor gets employees to work together as a team	1	2	3	4	5	6	7
c. My supervisor really tries to get our ideas about things	1	2	3	4	5	6	7
d. My supervisor lives up to his/her promises	1	2	3	4	5	6	7
e. My supervisor is fair in dealing with me	1	2	3	4	5	6	7

f. My supervisor is friendly toward
    employees   1   2   3   4   5   6   7
g. My supervisor lets me do my job
    without always looking over my
    shoulder   1   2   3   4   5   6   7

You have now completed the questionnaire. Please check to make sure you have answered all questions. Thank you.

Appendix C

Financial Work Sheet

While arranging some of the financial aspects of your organization, it is helpful to develop figures from a conservative, moderate, and optimal point of view.

Program/Service Descriptions

Conservative:

Moderate:

Optimal:

	Conservative	Moderate	Optimal
CAPITAL EQUIPMENT			

OPERATING EXPENSES:
Salaries/wages
Payroll taxes
Rent
Equipment maintenance
Utilities
Maintenance
Office supplies
Printing
Telephone
Postage
Travel
Marketing
Insurance
Legal/accounting
Staff development

Consultants
Education programming

	Conservative	Moderate	Optimal
INCOME:			
Membership assessment			
Program income			
Contracts			
Grants			
Other			

Operating Procedures
of MHEC Executive Committee

On September 29th the executive committee met to discuss selected questions on policy- and decision-making processes for the Manchester Health Education Consortium. After lengthy discussion, the committee voted to accept this summary as a statement of the project's operating procedures.

Summary Statement

The executive committee requested that it be vested with final decision-making authority in all matters pertaining to the grant and that this authority be granted by the Educational Council of NEHA. NEHHF, however, will act as the fiscal agent responsible for administering project funds.

Summary of Decisions on Procedural Questions

1. *Who decides on budget changes? Major policy changes?*
   The executive committee, within the framework of the decision- and policy-making procedures outlined below.
2. *Who is responsible for preparing minutes of the executive committee?*
   The MHEC director, or his designate, for the chairman of the executive committee.
3. *Who has the final decision to hire and/or fire various project personnel?*
   Refer to Summary Statement.
4. *Which decisions do administrators want to make? Be consulted on? Be informed of after the decision is made?*
   All policy and program decisions that pertain to budgetary matters, the commitments of the project and individual institutions, changes in the objectives and scope of the grant, and the hiring and firing of project personnel will be made by the executive committee. Project staff will inform the committee of all decisions made and actions taken.
5. *How will the group know when it has arrived at a decision?*
   By majority vote of a quorum of members present.
6. *What decisions of the executive committee on the project will be binding on individual hospitals?*
   All decisions except those which compromise or are in conflict with the principles or policies of individual institutions or those which increase the commitment of participating institutions beyond that already given.
7. *Does the committee expect to adopt a set of operating procedures or by-laws? Elect officers?*

This agreement is intended as a statement of operating procedures until such time as changes or additions are necessary. The executive committee will have two officers: chairperson and secretary-treasurer.

8. *Who decides what items go on the agenda? How will it be done?*
   All members and staff may submit agenda items. The director will prepare and distribute agendas, in consultation with the chairperson.

9. *What happens if a decision of the executive committee conflicts with the policy or needs of the New England Hospital and Health Foundation, Inc.?*
   The executive committee will decide on an issue-by-issue basis within the framework of this agreement.

10. *Should third parties from individual hospitals (for example, educators, department heads) or outside agencies (for example, universities) be brought into any decisions? Which ones? How?*
    The executive committee will solicit input from interested parties on an as-need basis. It is a policy of MHEC to seek maximum input on major decisions.

11. *What role should the project's education advisory group play in decision making?*
    This group, comprised of educators, will work with MHEC staff and make recommendations through it to the executive committee.

12. *Should anyone else be involved in the committee?*
    This item is tabled for later discussion pending efforts to expand project to other health organizations.

13. *Do we always need face-to-face meetings to make joint decisions or can we use such techniques as telephone polling?*
    Those decisions requiring prompt action between regularly scheduled meetings or concerning single-item matters can be made by telephone polling. Members will decide whether formal meetings are necessary.

14. *Who approves purchase of major equipment or services (such as audiovisual systems, management development programs, and so on)?*
    MHEC staff will approve those purchases clearly identified in the grant and budget. Major purchases, such as audiovisual systems or those having a major bottom-line impact, will be approved prior to purchase by the executive committee. NEHHF, Inc. will provide the executive committee with a monthly statement.

15. *What role will hospital trustees play in decision making regarding the project? Medical staffs?*
    Individual administrators assume full responsibility for informing both parties.

16. *What role will NEHA directors play in project decision making?*
    Refer to Summary Statement.

17. *Who will set project priorities and objectives? How?*
    These decisions will be made by the executive committee and individual institutions as outlined in the development plan submitted by staff.

Appendix E

MHEC Policy on Confidentiality and Use of Information

The executive committee of the Manchester Health Education Consortium (MHEC) officially adopts this statement of policy regarding confidentiality and the use of information.

1. The executive committee will exercise final authority over the use and release of project information within the guidelines established below.

2. Information in the following categories will be treated as public and shared with the New England Hospital and Health Foundation, the New Hampshire Hospital Association, organizations formally participating in the consortium, and other parties working with MHEC:
   a. data describing staff development resources held by consortium members;
   b. data describing past, present, and future staff development programs;
   c. data describing the numbers and characteristics of health personnel involved in the project;
   d. data describing education and training needs, goals, priorities, and plans; and
   e. other similar information descriptive in nature.

3. Specific information in the following categories about individual institutions will be treated as confidential and not released by staff to other participating organizations and groups without prior authorization of the administrator:
   a. data describing organizational climate, employee attitudes, management problems, and similar factors;
   b. statistical data describing the operations or performance of participating organizations, such as turnover rates, absenteeism, JCAH surveys, and so on; and
   c. similar information describing the internal operations of any organization(s)

4. Within single institutions, the following policies will apply:
   a. Public information will be available to all employees on request.
   b. Confidential information will be available to the administrator, the internal planning group for staff development, the education staff, and others designated by the administrator.
   c. Any individual or group which provides information for a particular survey will receive feedback on the results of that survey.
   d. Confidential information given by individuals will be reported only in summary form (for example, "the majority of department heads stated that they have working relationships with the fiscal office").
   e. At no time will any individual be identified as the source of information.

5. Individual administrators will approve all diagnostic plans and determine what information will and will not be collected within their organization.

6. Project staff will schedule regular data feedback sessions to the administrators and others within the framework of these policies.

7. All individuals with access to information will adhere to these policies.

8. The project evaluator(s) will have access to whatever information they need to do their jobs.

9. The executive committee and individual administrators will decide what information will be disseminated to outside parties, for example, project reports, journal articles, and so on.

Used with permission of Health Education Consortium, Inc.